FROM WONDERLAND TO CANCERLAND

A Young Woman's Journey Living with Melanoma

Sarah Toller

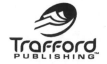

Trafford
PUBLISHING™

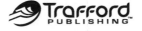

www.trafford.com

North America & international
toll-free: 1 888 232 4444 (USA & Canada)
phone: 250 383 6864 ♦ fax: 812 355 4082
email: info@trafford.com

This book is dedicated to
all those living with malignant melanoma
and their caregivers.

Hopes and dreams are just an illusion; all we have is the present.
— Sarah Toller

Table of Contents

A NOTE FROM SARAH'S MOM

I don't know why Sarah started writing her blog almost two years after diagnosis; I only learned of it by accident about three months before her death. And then I chose not to raise the subject because she said in the blog that it wasn't time for me to know about it. I do know, based on the many comments her postings elicited, that she touched the hearts of many people, and made numerous online friends from around the world. I am personally very thankful to have this record of her experience.

Shortly after Sarah died, several people approached me independently suggesting that her blog be made into a book with the hope that it could provide some perspective and advice to others travelling the same path, from someone who has "been there". While everyone's experience (mentally, emotionally and physically) with melanoma is different, it is my hope that Sarah's story will provide some information and guidance with regard to navigating our health care system, and some solace in knowing that others have gone before and ultimately found peace.

So here it is. I decided not to include any of the many supportive comments received on Sarah's blog as it would be difficult to obtain permission, and there were far too many to print. To everyone who supported Sarah on her journey (family, friends, co-workers, blogger buddies, and lurkers, too), I sincerely thank you. You did make a difference.

Also, sincere thanks to those who assisted, advised, and encouraged me. You know who you are. Most especially, I want to thank Derek Kaskiw, Sarah's "bestest friend", lover and husband, who unfailingly provided strength, encouragement, comfort and support to Sarah throughout her journey. No one knew how to care for Sarah as much as he did. He was, and I suspect probably still is, her rock.

This book contains the complete text of Sarah's blog almost verbatim, including profanities and angry rants. Grieving for one's own life is fraught with emotion.

Square brackets [ ] are used where I have added text for clarification, or to explain an acronym. Unfortunately, I had to delete some images due to print quality issues and copyright concerns. Also, since the names of Sarah's many doctors are not relevant to her story, they have been replaced with a letter that has no resemblance their name, e.g., the first doctor mentioned is referred to as Dr. A, the second doctor as Dr. B, etc.

Many websites are referenced in this book and were active at time of writing.

All profits from this book will be donated to registered Canadian charitable organizations that are currently researching treatments and cures for malignant melanoma, or providing support services to melanoma patients and caregivers.

Pat Best – May 2008

Que Sarah, Sarah[1]
Just an average chick living a new normal somewhere between Wonderland and Cancerland.

MAY 18, 2006

SOMETHING ABOUT SARAH

Well, I can't believe I'm doing this.

I think I need a place to vent, and possibly anonymous ears to listen to me.

My first post is going to be some background on my medical situation, copied and pasted from *www.mpip.org*, where I sometimes hang out to get info and not feel so alone in this.

I was diagnosed with stage 3 malignant melanoma (unknown primary) at the age of 27. Malignant melanoma is the deadliest skin cancer, and the most common cause of cancer death in women age 25 – 30, believe it or not. Here's how it all came about:

July 2004: Have a bit of pain in right arm. Feels like 10 bees stinging me at once deep inside my arm. Thought I pulled something at gym.

August 2004: Still have same occasional pain but not worried in the least. I'm enjoying my summer and playing soccer. Have tons of energy, working full time and going to school. Moving at end of August.

Early Sept 2004: I get out of shower and notice a golf-ball sized

---

1   Sarah's blog title. Her original blog is available at *http://que-sarah-sarah. blogspot.com/*

lump under right axilla [armpit and surrounding area]. Must have popped up virtually over night because it was summer and I was frequently shaving so would have noticed. I had a bad cold so I thought it was a reaction. Never really known anyone to have cancer so I had no idea that a swollen mass in armpit could be a big warning.

Sept 13, 2004: Went to family doctor who prescribed amoxicillin. Said the only time she has ever seen something like that is with mono [infectious mononucleosis]. Since I had mono at 15 that was not a possibility. I didn't perceive her to be concerned and I was still not concerned at all. I was so far removed from considering that it might be cancer that I even did an Arnold [Schwarzenegger] impression and said to her "As long as it's not a tooma."[2]

She looked at me funny but didn't say anything. That moment haunts me now... she knew it looked like a tumour. How mortifying and awkward.

One week later, Sept 2004: Lump not going down. Maybe it is bigger? Family doc says I need to consult a surgeon. It would be another week or so before I realized that meant "surgical oncologist". Lump is really starting to HURT and I have to be really careful with my arm because of the nerves being pinched. My doc can't get me in with a surgeon in London [Ontario] for at least a month so she says to go to emergency.

Late Sept 2004: I go to emerg and get an ultrasound of right axilla. I'm still CLUELESS! I thought maybe at worst it was a cyst and I'd need surgery. Doc says it is a lymph node but they don't know why. After a breast exam he says matter-of-factly "I'm pretty sure it is not breast cancer as there is no palpable mass in the breast."

That is the first time the "C" word is mentioned and I thought it was rude of him to be so matter of fact. He says I need to see a surgeon for a biopsy. I'm still not concerned... I've had a few biopsies before and they are a standard way to rule things out. As

---

2 Sarah-ism meaning "tumour"

I'm leaving, the nurse says "good luck!" and that rings in my ear. She knew.

Sept 24, 2004: I finally get a biopsy scheduled after returning to emerg for a second time with a note from my family doctor. Seems there aren't enough surgeons in this city and the wait is infinite to see one if you don't already have a diagnosis. So, the emerg doc has a friend who is a radiologist and he agreed to do the needle aspiration on the 27th as a favour to his buddy. Thank God!

Sept 27, 2004: Fine needle aspiration by Dr. A at South Street campus of London Health Sciences. He hints it might be lymphoma and says that it is highly treatable so not to worry. Also says it could be a number of other things including cat scratch disease [a bacterial illness characterized by chills, slight fever, and swelling of the lymph glands, often in the armpit]. Now I know it could be cancer. The panic sets in.

Sept 29, 2004: Dr. A calls with results. Looks like melanoma. His voice was very grave and sullen and I knew this was not good. I say "that's not a good one to have" as I choke back the tears and he says "No, it's not", and then I think he was trying to reassure me when he added "Sometimes bad things happen to good people." I took that as a death sentence.

Early October 2004: Meet with surgical onc [oncologist], Dr. B at the London Regional Cancer Centre. Says primary would have to be on trunk or right arm for it to drain to right axilla. There is nothing suspicious. Nine years earlier I had a mole removed from mid back but path [pathology report] came back clear. I showed onc the path report and he said that it would be very unlikely that it was that mole because of its characteristics and the fact that it was 9 years earlier. I still wonder. But it doesn't matter at this point.

Oct 14, 2004: Surgery to remove [lymph] nodes. Later found out 2 positive nodes lumped together in an ugly mass the size of a softball. Dr. B says it is better than he thought which surprised me. I didn't realize how bad he thought it was. I have drain in for about 4 days.

I do exercises and arm heals up great. Lost all feeling in armpit and some back of arm and breast. No biggie. Gotta be careful when I shave!

Mid Nov 2004: Start high dose interferon. That is the only option in Canada besides doing nothing. I didn't research the drug, I just trusted the onc. I was extremely fatigued most days, but some days I was mediocre. After 2 weeks, I asked to go on Paxil because the interferon was making me really negative. I thought about death and dying constantly and couldn't take it. I was teary all the time. After a few days on Paxil, I could see the light again. Interferon disturbed my thinking and cognitive abilities more than anything. The "flu-like" symptoms were negligible.

Dec 17, 2004: High dose treatment done. I get a break from treatment over Christmas and New Years! I felt 100% back to myself 3 days after treatment ended! I have just enough time to get my Christmas shopping done.

Early January 2005: Six weeks of radiation to right axilla. Tolerated this fine. Had about 2 weeks of pain while it oozed and healed. I am impressed with how well my skin has healed.

February 23, 2005: First low dose injection [of interferon]. Five hours after injection, the symptoms start and last 8 hours. I am in pure agony from the body aches, chills, migraine and fever of 104. Tylenol did not help in the least. I didn't know pain could be so painful!

February – April 15, 2005: Shots are going great. Much better than I expected. The first night was the worst by a mile. I take my shots on Sunday, Tuesday and Thursday nights. The Tylenol prevents any pain from creeping up. I say that some days I'm 80% myself and some days I'm 60% myself. I go for short walks for some exercise but definitely could not go to the gym! The fatigue is definitely there all the time and sometimes I just lay on the couch all day. Generally though, I can go out and about and be almost normal. I'm off the Paxil and have not had further depression issues. My appetite is fine and I have no change in taste. People are surprised at how "good" I look. I won't be playing soccer this year and I'm really sad about that! I'm not attempting to work because I can't predict when I'm going to feel good and when I'm not. I don't want the guilt nor the pressure of trying to work when I feel crappy. Also, my thinking has slowed down and I am very scatter-brained and have a short attention span. I think this break of 1.5 years from work will allow me to really get in touch with myself. I am excited about the possibilities. I've taken up yoga and am reading a lot of "self-help" books. I want to get my life back on track!

April 15, 2005: I get up nerve to ask my medical oncologist [Dr. C] a few scary questions. I never asked about staging but figured out on my own that I am stage 3, but because there was no primary, am I 3B or 3C? He says that he can't determine that but I am definitely not 3A, which I knew. I also asked about having children. He says I can go for it as soon as my cycles get back to normal after INF [interferon]. I have read that many oncs don't recommend pregnancy for stage 3. Dr. C believes the literature does not show a link between pregnancy and mm [malignant melanoma] recurrence. He says I have to live my life and if it is something that I want to do then I should. I'll wait at least 2 years I think.

Getting married on July 9th, 2005 to my love of 7 years, Derek. Dr. C said no problem to take 2 week break for INF so I can enjoy the wedding and honeymoon in Bermuda.

June 2005: Developed a bit of lymphedema and brachial plexopathy [an injured or disordered condition of the complex grouping of nerves supplying the chest, shoulder and arm] in right arm due to radiation. Not nice, but a small price to pay for my life.

August 2005: Transfer care to Princess Margaret Hospital in Toronto (two hours away) under Dr. D and Dr. E, after Dr. C leaves for Miami. I am very happy with PMH so far. They seem to have much more money and resources and get things done much faster.

Dec 2005: Decide to quit interferon at about 9/10 months. Current studies show that INF does not increase overall survival but it may add, on average, 12 months to your life. But, you feel like crap for 12 months too. Also, my docs feel that I likely got any benefit from the drug early on in treatment. It is the Christmas season and I want to feel good again. I really haven't kept track of exactly how many shots I took but I took a 2 week break in May and a 3 week break in July due to my wedding so I think that makes it about 9 or 10 months that I was on INF.

Dec 22, 2005: LOCAL RECURRENCE detected on my own! I am shocked. Located in what is still considered my right axillary node basin but it is really just beneath my collar bone and 1 cm out of my previous field of radiation! Surgery is scheduled for January 19th. Wait times are ridiculous. CT [scan] confirms no further mets [metastases]. This tumour has grown just like the previous. It went from nothing palpable to the size of a golf-ball virtually overnight and has now increased to the size of an apple in the 3 weeks since biopsy. I would say that is fast!

On a positive note, I feel 100% back to myself post-interferon except I have attention and memory difficulties.

Feb 20, 2006: Path results: 1 positive node. "Only" 5 cm, so smaller than I thought. Felt big because it was behind pec [pectoral] muscle. No further treatment (there is nothing in Canada). Appointments with onc every 3 months, CT scans every 6 months. 80% of stage 3C melanoma patients are dead within 5 years. Fuck that.

May 18, 2006: Still feeling fine. Back at work last week after 1.5 years off. Supplements I'm taking: Modified Citrus Pectin, Green Tea Extract, Turmeric. Crossing fingers and pleading with the universe. This was not supposed to happen.

posted by Sarah @ 7:23 PM   6 comments

OH BABY

Feeling a little melancholy today. Sad for what I've lost – they were only illusions anyway, so why am I so sad?

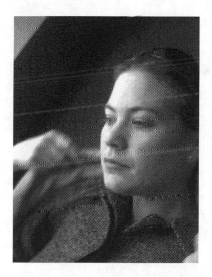

They say to picture what you want and work towards it. So that's what I've done. I did everything right. But then cancer came a knocking anyway. Fuck.

I feel like I'm in a dream, like none of this is real, but I know it is.

I'm sitting in our home office thinking about how perfect a little baby room it would be. But of course, my baby dreams are on hold indefinitely, probably permanently. I don't want to be pessimistic or fatalistic in my thinking, and I don't think I am. I think I'm realistic. I wanted to have a baby by now. Before Sept 2004 happened (the month where I got a rude awakening – I cannot control my destiny entirely, contrary to what Oprah has always taught me...) I was on a path. Get Derek and me permanent, stable jobs. Start saving for a house. Get pregnant. So I should be pregnant RIGHT NOW! Instead I have to somehow figure out how to live and move forward when the statistics say I will be dead within 5 years. What the fuck? I cannot wrap my mind around it. And I feel so good. It seems so unbelievable to me that tomorrow I could find a new lump, that I could have a seizure because the cancer spread to my brain, that I could cough up blood because it spread to my lungs. I have to live in the present now.

Living in the present. Isn't that what all the yogis and Buddhists and granola crunchers strive for so hard? I'll tell ya how to do it. Get cancer. Get a cancer with a bad prognosis. I can no longer picture past 3 months in the future. It's like I have become incapable of imagining it. I think it is too painful to imagine the future anymore. When your dreams are shattered with one phone call, you don't set yourself up for that pain again. It is (ironically) self preservation of sorts. Some more judgmental minds would say I'm setting myself up to die then. I have to envision being OK or there is no way I will be. It's all about positive attitude they say. To that I retort: BULL SHIT. If that were the case, then I never would have gotten cancer in the first place. Shit happens. Face it.

I can HOPE for the best, and God knows I do. But I cannot predict the future. My best indication lies in the stats on what has happened to the overwhelming majority of people in my exact situation. Sure, I can be the one that makes it! I WANT TO BE! But please tell me how to wrap my mind around the uncertainty of not knowing this for sure. I will live in limbo, not knowing, for the rest of my life! It's not like in 5 years, they can say I'm "all clear". There is no cure. It can come back at any time. I just don't know how to make the adjustment from living life knowing that I would probably live to 80, to knowing that I will probably be dead within a few years. It changes EVERYTHING.

Work for instance. After 1.5 years off for surgery, chemo, radiation, then more surgery, I am back at work on a part-time basis. I don't hate my job. It's fine. Do I love it? No. Would I love any job given the fact that life has become so incredibly precious to me in the last year? No. I don't want to work. Spending 8 hours a day "earning a living" is not how I want to live if I am indeed going to die soon. I've fucking earned a living! I want to do whatever the fuck I want to do every second of every fucking day. It's easier to go to work and suck it up when you know the odds are in your favour to live till you're 80. There is plenty of time for "free time". And don't come back at me with the old "well, you could get hit by a bus tomorrow...". That's a load of crap. Sure it could happen. But you know damn well that there is a 99.9% chance it won't and a 99.9% chance you'll live till 80. So every decision you make in life is based on that implicit understanding. You don't think about it often, but this knowledge is the basis for how you order and pace your life. You put off that trip to Europe so you can save for 3 years. You wait 10 years to have a child until you are "settled". You tell your mom you'll spend Christmas with her next year. I don't have the LUXURY of thinking that way anymore. Believe me I wish I did. It is much easier to live that way. Living in the present is not all it's cracked up to be.

My heart aches because I can't have a baby. The irresponsible, illogical part of me says, fuck it. Get pregnant and hope for the best. The realistic part of me says if I have a recurrence while pregnant I can't be treated. What if I die when the baby is new born? What if I leave Derek widowed with a 2 year old? Is that fair to him? To the child? And this whole thing would be even more traumatic than it already is for me if I found out I was terminal with a baby that I couldn't see grow up. I'd love to think that the universe wouldn't allow these things to happen if I had a baby. But I know it doesn't work that way. I've seen too many beautiful people, young, old, healthy, strong, mothers, daughters, fathers, sons, die of this disease (online friends) in the past year to believe that God would give me special treatment.

God. Do I believe in God? I believe in something but I don't know what. I'm agnostic I suppose. I don't believe that anything purposely gave me cancer or that I am being tested or that it is karma. I am an organism. Just like a cat gets cancer, I can too. Just like a bee gets swatted, I can too. Shit happens. It isn't my destiny. Shit just happens. I never thought it would really happen to me. Not now.

posted by Sarah @ 12:00 PM   2 comments

FOOD + CROQUET = GOOD TIMES

The summer is fun. Last summer I was afraid of the sun so I didn't much enjoy myself. I prayed for rain or cloud cover most days. Plus, I was on interferon (that's the chemo I was on for 11 months) so I was super tired and dazed most of the time.

Anyhoo[3], this summer is different. My second summer with melanoma (well, actually my third, but I was unaware it was growing inside me in Summer '04) and although I don't plan on baking at the beach, I also don't plan to let the sun ruin my summer. I have to be practical about it. The sun can do no more damage to my current state of affairs. It isn't going to make my disease progress. It could give me a second melanoma, and although my chances are slightly increased for this because I've had one, it is still unlikely. And even if I had a second primary down the road, I am so aware of my skin I'd definitely catch it early. Melanoma is 90% curable if caught early, before it spreads downwards into the lymph system and blood. I fear not a second melanoma. I fear the cancer that is already in me, because it is so advanced.

So, to celebrate the coming of summer, Derek and I held the First Annual Vegan Potluck and Croquet Tournament in our backyard on Saturday! Mmmmmm.... everyone brought delicious food. I made stuffed baked mushrooms with vegan cream cheese, onion and cilantro, a fiery Mexican bean salad, and roasted veggies. Others brought hummus, baba ganoush and pita, fattoush salad [Lebanese or Syrian type salad], an Asian noodle salad, fruit

---

3   Sarah-ism for "anyway"

11

salad marinated in booze and fruit kabobs. We have so much left over too, since no one felt like carrying their leftovers home.

The croquet tournament was a hoot. We had three heats. I was in an all girl heat and we totally sucked. The rule became, if it goes thru the wicket, over the wicket or beside the wicket, it counts because the game was getting too long. I laughed my butt off though, it was pure comedy. Ben was the grand champ of the tourney and his grand prize was a beach ball, bubbles and a New Kids On the Block hip-sack circa 1989 in its original packaging!

posted by Sarah @ 4:08 PM   0 comments

I RUN AND I RANT

Did I mention I run? Yup, it's a newish thing. Since February this year. Before cancer (B.C.), I was fairly active, going to the gym 3 times a week (or so) and playing soccer. But I always thought I couldn't run outside. I could run on the treadmill, but put me outside and I'd be breathless within a couple of minutes.

I went thru the whole cancer thang[4] and put on a few pounds from being a forced couch potato for a year, so in Feb I decided to get ready for bikini season. Even if I'm not going to be lying on the beach ever again, I can still have a great body, right? As an aside, it seems trivial and superficial to be focusing on body image in my situation, I know. But it is a) easier for me to focus on something that I can control with my body right now, and b) a testament to the fact that I value my body so much more now than I ever did. After being so sick from chemo for a year that I was often "too tired to speak" as I'd say, or too exhausted to walk from the couch to the kitchen to get a glass of water, I don't take for granted the fact that I have a strong body right now and I want to feel the power of it.

I want to run, to push it. Does that make sense? I want people to look at me and think, "She looks like a strong, healthy woman", and I want to feel that way about myself. For the most part I do. I don't think of myself as a cancer patient. That's not me. I am strong and healthy. The cancer part does not fit and it won't become part of my identity. I know that has sort of been the focus of my blog so far, but I think that's why I needed to start this. To

---

4   Sarah-ism for "thing"

give that small piece of me a voice, to get it off my chest here so it doesn't invade my life.

But I digress. I started the "Couch to 5k" program in Feb and it has worked wonders for me physically. So, today I had an awesome run. I've decided to push it a bit more by going longer distances. My technique will be the 10 and 1, where you run for 10 and walk for 1 over and over. Today I did three 10 minute runs. Sweet. I think I'll do that for a week then push it up to 11 and 1 and so on.

In other cancer related news, I had my 1 year follow-up at the lymphedema clinic today. I have mild lymphedema in my right arm from the surgeries and radiation. It sucks, but it could be much worse. Apparently I have had a 13% increase in size since last June. That's not cool. I asked about Kenisio tape and the nurse told me she has never heard of it. Are you kidding me? That's why I transferred my care to Toronto [in addition to medical oncologist's move to Miami]. The nurse in the lymphedema clinic at the London [Regional] Cancer Centre didn't even know what Kinesio tape was. I called my Toronto hospital and apparently they have someone who treats with this method for free. But lo and behold, it is a trial and only open to breast cancer patients.

Um, I will rant a bit now. I know there is no cure for breast cancer. But it's like our society has forgotten that many other cancers exist. Sure, 1 in 8 women will get breast cancer, but more will get some other form of cancer! 1 in 2 of us will get cancer. Do the math. Yet everywhere I go it is pink ribbon this, pink ribbon that. It would be great, if only other cancers got the same support and funding from the public.

Breast cancer awareness and funding is this huge machine now. The more we hear about it, the more people give money to it, the more resources breast cancer patients get, but other cancer patients get left in the dust.

I've been told numerous times by doctors, nurses and social workers in the field that the topic is highly political and controversial in the cancer community. My local Wellspring [a network of cancer support centres] only has support groups for breast cancer patients for instance. Um, hello? Why? We all have scars, we all have body image issues, we all stay awake at night wondering if we are going to live or die. Why do the breast cancer patients get the support? Probably because someone died and left money to fund a breast cancer support group. Why can't I get into the Kinesio trial, even though my lymph node dissection of the axilla and radiation is the exact same reason breast cancer patients develop lymphedema too? Because breast cancer has the funding for research. Melanoma doesn't. I just hope they find a cure for breast cancer soon so the rest of us can be helped too.

My request is that if you are thinking about donating to breast cancer, maybe think about donating to something more broad that allocates money to many different cancers. Enough with the pink food processors and quarters already. Support other cancer foundations as well!

Canadian Melanoma Foundation
Melanoma Research Foundation
Canadian Cancer Society

posted by Sarah @ 9:29 PM   3 comments

FIVE FOOT SIX ABOVE

Fuck. The irony. I'm watching the final episodes of Six Feet Under on DVD yesterday, poking and prodding my armpit like I always do, and I find a fucking lump! It never ceases to amaze me that when I find this shit, I am doing the most benign activities, thinking the most benign thoughts, feeling supremely healthy and enjoying life. Out of nowhere this shit happens, I tell ya.

OK, it might not be a recurrence. I hope to God it isn't. I'm not going to get worked up too much either way. I know I can't know. The myth that one knows when something is wrong with the body is utter shit. I never know. When I present with symptoms to my onc and am convinced I have brain mets, I don't. When I present with a lump that I'm convinced is nothing, it is. I have no fucking clue. All I know is this new lump, a bit smaller than a pea, was not there a few days ago. I see my onc on Tuesday.

It can't be a cancerous lymph node because they have all been taken out. The radiation was supposed to prevent recurrences in that area too. That's why I'll be floored if it is. But, then, I guess because I had a recurrence outside the field of radiation in December, that could have spread to the area which was previously treated. Could this be a sub-q [subcutaneous] tumour? Damn it.

Think positive. Think positive. Think positive.

I just can't fathom what else it would be. Fuck Fuck Fuck!

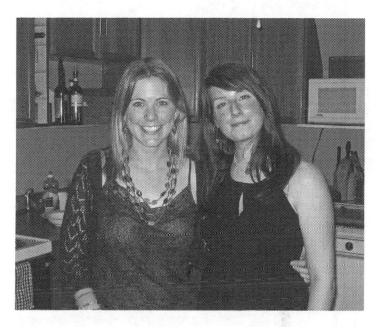

On a lighter note, here's a pic of me this past weekend looking like a total LOSER (but healthy as shit I must say!) with my friend before we went out to a bachelorette party. I swear, my bra didn't show through my shirt, it is just because of the flash on the camera! Ha ha ha!

posted by Sarah @ 3:34 PM   4 comments

THE PROPHET

I walk up to the counter at the liquor store today holding two bottles of wine and the older gentleman behind the counter greets me with, "My dear, are you old enough to drink?". I am a bit taken aback, but flattered, and reply, "Yes, but I wish I wasn't – I'm 29", for lack of something wittier to say. He pauses, smiles, and says, "Ah, you haven't even reached your best years.... Your 30s and 40s will be the best."

Could he be some kind of prophet? In any case, I needed to hear that today.

posted by Sarah @ 7:56 PM 0 comments

EDUCATION AND PREVENTION

Imogen Potter was a beautiful woman. I knew her from a cancer message board I belong to. She was only 37 when she died in May 2005.

Please take a moment to watch her video[5]. I'm sure wherever she is, she would be happy to know her message is still making an impact.

Here is a great video on how melanoma spreads[6]. People don't often understand how a tiny skin blemish can kill.

posted by Sarah @ 6:42 PM   0 comments

---

5   *http://www.bbc.co.uk/videonation/articles/b/birmingham_livingwithcancer.shtml*

6   *http://www.mayoclinic.com/health/cancer/MM00638*

WAITING TO EXHALE

Spent last 2 days in Toronto seeing different doctors about my lump.

My medical onc felt what I felt, and also thought he felt something else. Gulp. I felt what he felt and was pretty sure that was just scar tissue from prior surgeries. But I'm not a doctor, just a know-it-all.

Today I had two FNAs (Fine Needle Aspirations) which is where they stick a needle in the lump(s) to draw junk (yes, that's the medical term) out to biopsy. God bless Princess Margaret Hospital as they can draw the fluid, and read the slide and get an answer in 5 minutes! He said he could only see blood cells in the sample which is AWESOME but he took one more sample and I'll get the results Friday. Derek's mouth was open in awe during the whole thing, he was so intrigued by the process. I don't think he was grossed out, he was just utterly amazed at what the doctors were doing.

The tiny lump I found is so small that it could barely be aspirated and he said that he can't be 100% sure it isn't cancerous because the sample was so small. So, I have an appointment with my surgical onc on Friday for a consult and from there we'll make an appointment to get the sucker out and it can be biopsied better. Third surgery to my poor armpit in a year and a half.

I also had a CT scan which will show if there are any tumours anywhere else in my body. Results likely Friday from my surgeon. That's the really scary one. Please don't be in any organs!!

So, there is hope! This could be a false alarm.

We also scored free tickets to Cronenberg's Andy Warhol exhibit at the Art Gallery of Ontario (AGO) and when we return this weekend to the T-dot [short form for Toronto] we'll get to check that out. We have a very fun 1st anniversary weekend planned in Toronto, I just hope we get some great news to kick it off with otherwise it'll be hard to enjoy the weekend.

Here's a wedding pic of us because we're so cute! July 9, 2006 will be one year! How did that happen? In fact, where did the last 8.5 years we've been together go!

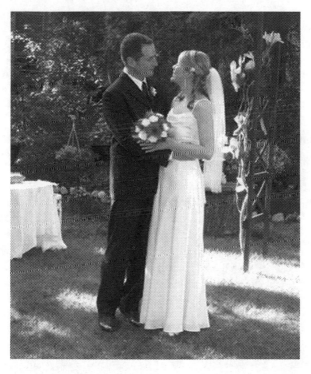

He's my bestest friend and it breaks my heart he has to go thru this shit with me.

posted by Sarah @ 8:27 PM   2 comments

WAITING TO FULLY EXHALE

We had a wicked weekend in Toronto. Lotsa shopping, lotsa eating at my fave vegan restaurant, Fressen[7], a fun laid-back wedding reception for some friends that eloped, lotsa walking and reminiscing, "When we lived in Toronto...". I lived in downtown TO for 5 years, and the D-man [Derek] lived there for 2. We miss it, but have made a life 2 hours outside where life is slower and the houses are much cheaper.

Still in the dark on what is going on in my armpit. I only got partial results from my CT [scan] on Friday because the analysis of my whole body wasn't in. My lungs are clear – huge sigh of relief because I've been having some chest pain but I will now 100% attribute that to nerve damage and healing from surgeries and radiation. Some activity in my right axilla. The tiny lump that I found is too small to light up, but there is a bigger area that is unusual compared to my last CT in December. That would be the area that my onc felt and that the FNA said was clear (twice). My surgeon feels it is likely scar tissue seeing as the FNA's were negative and the fact that my last CT was prior to my last surgery. It makes sense that the area would be bulkier. But, to be sure I have to have an MRI of the area.

Wait time rant. My MRI isn't scheduled till July 21st at 12:15 am, and that is in a city 2 hours away from me. My surgeon implied that it would be done this week, but I think she is slightly out of touch with the reality of medical imaging wait times. Of

---

7   Fressen, 478 Queen St. Toronto, ON 416-504-5127

course, the CT was done in near record time, but a CT only takes 5 minutes, whereas an MRI takes 45 minutes or so.

So, the jury is still out. And it will be out for another 2 weeks. Boo.

My surgery can't be scheduled till after the MRI, but I know there will be surgery. It will just be a matter of it being minor to remove the tiny lump to see what it is, or major to remove the other mass too. My surgeon indicated that if this other mass is malignant, the surgery will be riskier than my prior two because there is only scar tissue and nerves and arteries left in that area, no fatty tissue so she might opt not to do it. Um, what? I'll be shopping for another surgeon if she does take that stand, but we'll cross that bridge if we get to it. I'm 80% confident it is scar tissue. Trying desperately to get a surgery date for ASAP after the July 21st MRI but no one will return my calls from the surgeon's office. Last time I needed surgery in December, the secretary was on vacation so no one booking dates with the surgeon and my surgery was a month after diagnosis. I know I'm looking at at least a month from initially finding lump, to surgery this time too. The waiting is sometimes the worst part of all this.

I took this week off work. I am "in training" in my new position, which basically means reading tax legislation at my desk for 7.25 hours/day. As if I can concentrate at my desk when I have this shit on my mind. It would be another story if I had actual work to do, but it is hard enough to keep my eyes open reading that stuff on a good day so I said screw it for this week.

I think I may go in next week for the 3 days I'm supposed to work and suck it up. I'm still on a gradual back-to-work rehab program (topped-up from my insurance company for the days I'm not there) which makes it pretty flexible for me to just not come in if I don't feel I'm physically or emotionally up for it. This week off is just to remain sane. Physically I feel 100%. Must go for run tonight and get back on track with that!

posted by Sarah @ 1:36 PM   0 comments

WWW.GOVEG.COM[8]

I often wonder if people wonder to themselves if my veganism is the reason I have cancer. The thought must cross their minds right? I'm usually one of the only vegans they know, and I'm usually the only person under 40 they've ever met with cancer. So I can see if they might make that a connection.

Maybe no one does. But I can see why people would, if they do. People need to find reasons to believe this sort of thing could never happen to them.

Anyway, I just want to say: If that has crossed your mind then lay it to rest and come up with another theory as to why this happened to me and not you.

I have met hundreds of cancer survivors online and in person in the past year and a half, many of them my age and younger, and I believe I am the only vegan in the mix. There is no correlation. In fact, many people switch to a plant-based diet based on their own research or on the advice of nutritionists after a cancer diagnosis because cancer rates tend to be lower in people that adopt this lifestyle. Of course, this is not a rule. Anyone can get cancer.

I am pretty confident that my primary lesion was a mole I had removed when I was 18, a full year before I even became vegetarian.

Just had to get that off my chest.

posted by Sarah @ 10:42 PM   0 comments

---

8   The website *www.goveg.com* includes health and ethical reasons to become vegetarian, vegetarian and vegan recipes, and much more. Check it out.

A LITTLE DENIAL WITH THOSE FRIES?

All this waiting has not been so bad. The little lump in my armpit doesn't bother me so I am able to pretend it isn't there. Or pretend to pretend it isn't there. The big lump, I have convinced myself that, yes, it is definitely scar tissue. The MRI on Thursday is just a technicality. It is to prove what I already know.

I'm getting good at lying too. My parents think I've been at work. My dad thinks I went to Toronto mid week last week to see a concert (so what if the concert was actually Friday). When people ask how things are going or when my next Dr.'s appt. is I tell them everything is great and I have an appt. every 3 months and a CT scan every 6. I'm not due for another check-in for a while still, everything is fine!

I've told a couple of friends but that's it besides the anonymous internet community. I just can't bring myself to crush people's hopes and expectations, especially if this is a false alarm. I'm planning on waiting until I have the results back from my surgery to tell anyone. If they are bad, I'll have to tell. If they are fine, no one needs to know I just went thru a month of uncertainty.

I sometimes think it is probably more painful for family and friends to watch me go through this stuff than it is for me. It's not because of the way they act or react, it is because I know how I would feel if it were someone close to me. It would be torture not being able to help, not knowing what to say, not being able to solve the problem, to watch me in pain or in emotional turmoil. Worse to be the caregiver than the patient I think.

Obviously this has been hard for me. But the brain is a miraculous thing. Able to adapt, able to persevere. And if all else fails, there are always drugs that make everything seem A-OK! A little Valium with those fries?

Life goes on as usual, and I love it! It is such a cliché, but you really do appreciate things more once you experience something like this. In a lot of ways, life is sooooo much more fun than it was for the first 27 years of my life, because now my eyes are finally fully open. Cheesy. But so true.

Today, sitting on the back deck, I was startled by a little birdie that zipped in out of nowhere and landed right by my feet. Silly little baby birdie was learning how to fly and flew right into the after-dinner coffee party of 6 big human predators. He must have been so scared. After about 30 seconds, he got himself together enough to scramble off the deck and onto the lawn. The next half hour was quite entertaining watching mama and papa cardinal encouraging little tweety to fly.

Poor little guy kept flying into the wood fence because he couldn't get up high enough. Luckily, he eventually figured out that he could just crawl underneath and into the next yard. I hope he got back to the nest OK. It really was amazing to see how Mr. and Mrs. C communicated and demonstrated to Baby C. It reminded me of a parent teaching their child to ride a bike. We really are so similar. If I was actually on Valium right now I might end this entry by asking philosophically, we're all just one aren't we?

posted by Sarah @ 10:20 PM   1 comments

GOOD VIBES NEEDED

MRI was last Thursday at 12 am, 2 hours from home. Gah.

My sweet friend Liz came with me and waited the 45 minutes while I was strapped to a plank with velcro right up to my head and put into the cavernous machine that clangs and bangs the whole time while it is supposedly taking detailed images of my insides. Fun times.

I'm claustrophobic and took a Clonazepam to take the edge off then closed my eyes tight and deep breathed the entire time. Once about a year ago, I ran out of an MRI in hysterics before the procedure even started. Luckily now I've developed a technique to get through it.

It was a close one though. The technician had to reconfigure the bed because I refused to get into the cage contraption that was set up. They like to put a cage over your head so you can't move. I. Can. Not. Do. That. For freaks like me, they have this other, less than ideal device, that comes up sort of like a shield over your face, but not over your eyes. He was very kind and understanding and set the thing up especially for me.

So, tomorrow I suppose I'll get the results of the MRI. They want to find out if the big mass in my armpit that my oncs feel but 2 FNAs say is negative for cancer is indeed just scar tissue. Right. It fucking better be.

I'm definitely getting the little lump that has become more worrisome excised tomorrow. I say more worrisome, because in the 3.5 weeks I've waited since I first found the lump, to when I saw my medical onc, to when I saw my surgical onc, to when

I finally have an appt. to get it removed, it has grown. Before, it was definitely smaller than a pea. Now, it is definitely larger than a pea. Boo.

Please send your positive vibes my way tomorrow! I'm still hoping for a miracle! Maybe it is just a pea growing inside me! Heck, we planted some in the garden this summer, who's to say a seed didn't implant in me?

posted by Sarah @ 8:47 PM   0 comments

GOOD NEWS, BAD NEWS

Big mass is scar tissue.

Small mass is highly suspicious for recurrent melanoma. Removed today. Pathology will make final call. I'll get the results sometime within 2 weeks. Not that it really matters. There isn't much else it could be.

I was awake for the whole procedure and the surgeon showed me the small mass she removed. Looked so harmless.

Anyway, it's been a long day and I don't feel like talking about this shit. I'm soooo tired of it. I'd say I'm over it, but I can't be. Wish I could snap my fingers or press rewind.

No further treatment. As I've said before, there is no adjuvant treatment [additional treatment following surgery] beyond what I've already done and that didn't work. Now we just cherry pick tumours and hope they don't spread to organs.

It is such a weird feeling to be incredibly disappointed in your body but incredibly grateful for it at the same time. My body is doing a wonderful job at keeping the disease in the same local area. For that I am so grateful. But, I am still so dismayed at the fact that a) I ever got this in the first place, and b) that I wasn't one of the people that go recurrence free for years and years or the rest of their lives.

So many people I have met online have been diagnosed after me and are already dead. I think of those people daily and remember how lucky I am really. I am here now. No one is guaranteed more than this second. I will not waste time wallowing in self-pity. If I allow the cancer to destroy my experience of today and my spirit, then it has already won. I know this will never happen. I can't conceive that I could ever take a second of my life for granted again.

posted by Sarah @ 9:20 PM   3 comments

JULY 30, 2006, 12:56 AM

CAMPING

Just so ya know, my arm feels good. I literally have zero pain from the incision because of all the nerve damage from prior surgeries and radiation to my axilla. I'm sure she could have performed the excision without any anaesthesia as the whole area is perma-numb.

Other benefits of having had prior radiation to the area are that I no longer sweat or grow hair in that armpit! Think of all the dollars I have saved on razors and deodorant because I'm only using half as much!

Notice my right arm in the shots of me doing terrible yoga poses on the beach. It is clearly bigger than my left arm from the elbow up. That is what mild lymphedema looks like.

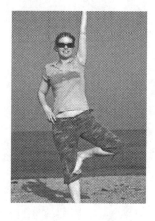
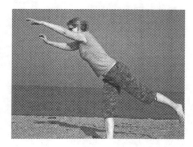

Went camping Friday night at Rondeau Provincial Park[9] with a girlfriend. It was supposed to be 2 nights, but our other friend was sick so she had to cancel. Liz and I decided just to stay one night so we could come back home and spend the second night with the sicky-poo watching movies. Plus, there was a 60% chance of thunderstorms the second night. It was hot! And I was very greasy, sweaty, and all-around nasty as you can see from the pics!

posted by Sarah @ 12:56 AM   2 comments

---

9   For information about Rondeau Provincial Park go to
    http://www.ontarioparks.com/ENGLISH/rond.html

I THINK I KNEW THAT

According to this article[10], [entitled] The Psychological Challenges Facing Melanoma Patients [written by Andrew W. Kneier, PhD], I am coping with my diagnosis incredibly well. Interesting. I think I knew that. I'm pretty proud of myself.

posted by Sarah @ 5:50 PM   3 comments

---

10 *http://www.cancerlynx.com/challenge.html*

WHAT IS, IS

Have lots I want to write, it's just never the right time. I'm reading a fabulous book I wanna talk about.... but I can't be bothered tonight.

Work is keeping me busy, and tired. I got the 3 days/week rehab program extended "indefinitely". That basically means that I work 3 days instead of 5, do my job as per usual, get paid almost the same (God bless long-term disability insurance!) and have a lot less stress.

I've been having many post-interferon cognitive difficulties [that] are keeping me on part-time disability (will list these in a future post), and coupled with the fact that I perpetually need 10 – 11 hours sleep in order to function at what I still consider to be a sub-optimal level (never mind what happens to me on 7 – 8 hours sleep...train wreck!!). Oh, and stress. I don't generally feel stressed, but I also think that if I push myself to do too much too soon given the circumstances, then I am bound to crack and have a nervous breakdown... especially considering a wee past history of anxiety and depression. I have learned the hard way about how much I can handle on my plate at once. Let's just say I'm pretty sure my plate is full and I'm not hungry for more.

Side note: I have a prior history of anxiety and panic disorder. I find it incredibly ironic and psychologically intriguing, that since my diagnosis with cancer almost 2 years ago, I have not had one panic attack – not even upon receipt of that dreadful (and somewhat cliché) phone call that changed my life forever. Any amateur psychologists out there want to take a crack at that one? Maybe facing my worst fear has made all other illogical/irrational fears pale in comparison thus curing my anxiety? Now instead of many little fears, I just have one big one. And this one is a valid and real fear, not irrational. Cancer cured my anxiety disorder. But in others, I'm sure cancer caused their anxiety disorder. I've always gotta be different.

Still no path report to report. I will be harassing my oncologist's secretary again on Thursday (day off). I'm not waiting on the edge of my seat or anything though. It honestly doesn't matter too much if it was 100% a recurrence or not. What is, is. Nothing changes treatment wise for me so I'm not concerning myself too much with the details of the offending tissue's pathology. What matters is that it is out.

Rant of the Day: I was all set to join the gym across the street from my work today. They inform me that the membership is only $28/month... IF I sign up for a year in advance. So, I ask if there is a monthly membership fee and am informed that it is $60/month – extortion in my humble opinion, especially considering that this is a bare bones gym with minimal equipment, classes only offered over the lunch hour, and only 2 TVs that you can't even plug your headset into.

This really frustrates me, because my plan to stay in shape (OK, get back into shape) and use the fabulous equipment to get buns of steel was thwarted because of a little detail: I have a serious life-threatening illness and I can't commit to a year membership. Shit could change on a dime for me as I've witnessed twice since December already. I'm all for positive thinking but, come on, I have to be financially responsible too!

So, I walked out with a resolve to get back into running even though I'm pretty bored of it and was really looking forward to going back to the gym to change it up a bit.

None of my whining should negate the fact that I am EXTREMELY grateful to be in a place right now where I can contemplate physical pursuits and bitch about membership fees. I don't take this for granted for one second.

posted by Sarah @ 7:54 PM   0 comments

MY LOVE

My love. Thank you.

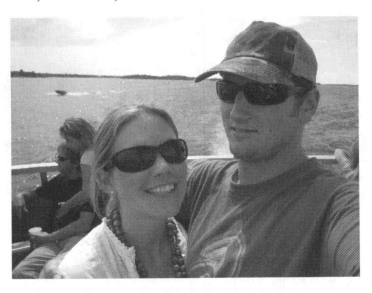

posted by Sarah @ 8:29 PM   0 comments

GRACE AND GRIT

I'm reading *Grace and Grit: Spirituality and Healing in the Life and Death of Treya Killam Wilber* by Ken Wilber and I am thoroughly enjoying it. Treya died of breast cancer in the early 90s and her husband was (is) a respected transcendental psychologist in the U.S. with several major publications on the subject. It is very interesting to read how they wrestled with modern medicine as well as eastern medicine and philosophies of illness during Treya's battle.

It is something that I have been wrestling with too, as there are so many mixed messages about illness in our society. On the one hand, we want to believe that if you are good and kind and "Positive", you can effectively beat any kind of illness or that, in fact, you will never become seriously ill in the first place. But the reality is that people get sick and there is no rhyme or reason to it and often nothing that can be done about the outcome. Healing is a word that is often misunderstood to mean "cure". Really, healing is about achieving a sort of inner grace and wisdom, a place of acceptance, an understanding of one's role within the world, and of the impermanence of everything.

I want to quote this book and share, because it really articulates well all the different messages we are given towards illness. No wonder I've felt so confused and have had such a hard time searching and finding meaning to my cancer.

From Grace & Grit:
... we had to face...dealing with the sickness of cancer, dealing

with all the various meanings and judgments that our different cultures and subcultures attached to this illness, that cloud of voices, images, ideas, fears, stories, photographs, advertisements, articles, movies, television shows...vague, shapeless, but dense, ominous... full of fear and helplessness...

And it wasn't just the general society at large that supplies various stories. Treya and I were exposed to several different cultures and sub-cultures, each of which had something very definite to say. Here are just a few:

1. Christian – The fundamentalist message: Illness is basically a punishment from God for some sort of sin. The worse the illness, the more unspeakable the sin.

2. New Age – Illness is a lesson. You are giving yourself this disease because there is something important you have to learn from it in order to continue your spiritual growth and evolution. Mind alone causes illness and mind alone can cure it. A yuppified post-modern version of Christian Science.

3. Medical – Illness is fundamentally a biophysical disorder, caused by biophysical factors (from viruses to trauma to genetic predisposition to triggering agent). You needn't worry about psychological or spiritual treatment for most illnesses because such alternative treatments are usually ineffectual and may actually prevent you from getting the proper medical attention.

4. Karma – Illness is the result of negative karma; that is, some non-virtuous past actions are now coming to fruition in the form of a disease. The disease is "bad" in the sense that it represents past nonvirtue; but "good" in the sense that the disease process itself represents the burning up and the purifying of the past misdeed; it's a purgation, a cleansing.

5. Psychological – As Woody Allen put it, "I don't get angry, I grow tumors instead." The idea is that, at least in pop psychology, repressed emotions cause illness. The extreme form: illness

is a death wish.

6. *Gnostic* — *Illness is an illusion. The entire manifest universe is a dream, a shadow, and one is free of illness only when one is free from illusory manifestation altogether, only when one awakens from the dream and discovers instead the one reality beyond the manifest universe. Spirit is the only reality, and in Spirit there is no illness. An extreme and somewhat off centered version of mysticism.*

7. *Existential* — *Illness itself is without meaning. Accordingly, it can take any meaning I choose to give it, and I am solely responsible for these choices. Men and women are finite and mortal, and the authentic response is to accept illness as part of one's finitude even while imbuing it with personal meaning.*

8. *Holistic* — *Illness is a product of physical, emotional, mental, and spiritual factors, none of which can be isolated from the others, none of which can be ignored. Treatment must involve all of these dimensions (although in practice this often translates into an eschewal of orthodox treatments, even when they might help).*

9. *Magical* — *Illness is retribution. "I deserve this because I wished So-and-so would die" Or, "I better not excel too much, something bad will happen to me." And so on.*

10. *Buddhist* — *Illness is an inescapable part of the manifest world; asking why there is illness is like asking why there is air. Birth, old age, sickness, and death — these are the marks of this world, all of whose phenomena are characterized by impermanence, suffering, and selflessness. Only enlightenment, in the pure awareness of nirvana, is illness finally transcended, because then the entire phenomenal world is transcended as well.*

11. *Scientific* — *Whatever the illness is, it has a specific cause or cluster of causes. Some of these causes are determined, others*

*are simply random or due to pure chance. Either way, there is
no "meaning " to illness, there is only chance or necessity.*

*Men and women necessarily and intrinsically swim in the ocean
of meaning; Treya and I were about to drown in it. On the way home
in the car, on that first day [after diagnosis], the various meanings
were already flooding through us, and nearly choking Treya.*

Those two pages of this book just made everything so much
clearer for me. It is like a weight has been lifted off my shoulders.
When you learn you are ill, or you learn that anyone is ill, you
automatically start searching for meaning or reasons why. Why
this happened to them as opposed to me. Why this happened to
me, and not them.

Before I got sick myself, I am ashamed to say, I would often
attribute others' misfortunes and illnesses to either #2 New-Age
(Oprah Winfrey has managed to brain-wash half of North America
into believing this crap), or #5, Psychological. Fair enough, in order to feel safe and secure in our own world and our own immor-
tality, we desperately seek to believe in a reason why bad things
happen to other people and how we can avoid bad things happening to us. It is human nature to seek out that comfort, it is the
same reason why I believe people subscribe to various religions.
Logic and reason are thrown to the wind because logic and reason
don't often make life feel comfy and cozy and like everything will
be A-OK or for the greater "good".

I have wrestled with the questions and the meaning. Am I being punished for something I did in this life? In a past life? Did
I somehow wish this upon myself by not appreciating my life
more? When I had a major depressive episode 6 years ago and
I fleetingly thought that death could be a decent alternative to
the mental torture I was going through, was this thought somehow coming true for me now? Are my emotions killing me? Did
I bottle up emotions to the point where they became a physical
illness? Have I not been positive enough? Did I not want to have
a future badly enough? Did I judge others too harshly? Did I take
the wrong path with my life and not realize that I was supposed
to take a different path? Is there some message a la Oprah Winfrey
I'm supposed to get out of this? If I figure out the message will I

be cured?

The answer to all these questions is clearly and logically, NO. And I have to remember that. My life has been great, is great, I am a good person, I have led a fairly healthy lifestyle, I have committed no (mortal) sins, and I don't believe I am being punished. Thinking that any being (such as God?) is punishing me or anyone [else] specifically is highly ego-centric. I can't fathom that out of the billions of living creatures on earth and in this universe, God would single me out to teach me some sort of lesson. Puh-leeze. Life is so much bigger than petty lessons in being a decent person or living an "authentic life" or finding one's "true calling". Fuck, I'm so mad at Oprah right now!

It is hard when society sends you so many mixed messages. But ultimately, I truly believe in a combination of the Medical, Scientific, Buddhist, and Existential models as outlined above. There is nothing I did to deserve this. And I accept that we are all mortal beings. Illness is not necessarily a "bad" thing. It is a part of life. And death is also a part of life, not the end of life. To live in constant fear of illness and death causes suffering. And I don't want to suffer as it ruins my experience of this moment, which as I've stated before, is all that we are guaranteed.

posted by Sarah @ 10:42 AM   1 comments

FREAKING OUT

I am freaking out. The following emails say it all. I can't
handle this shit. I just can't. I can't do this again. My heart is
breaking.

<u>Me</u>:

Hi Dr. Surgical Oncologist,

*Sorry to bother you directly. I have been calling your office for a
month now trying to get my path results from the excision you did
back on July 25th, without any luck.*

*I have requested that you call me multiple times, or that some-
one let me know what is happening. My calls are not returned and
when I do happen to reach your secretary directly she says she'll
call me back with info then doesn't. The one time she did return my
call, it was 2 weeks later and she wanted to book me for the excision! I had clearly left detailed messages that I had had an excision
and was looking for the pathology report.*

*I resorted to calling Dr. Medical Oncologist's secretary the week
before last and she is having no luck getting the info either. Dr.
M.O. called and left a message that there was no record of me having the excision at all.*

*Is the pathology not in yet? What has taken so long? When it is
found, can a copy please be sent to me at home?*

*I cannot be reached during the day this week but please do leave
a message on my answering machine or email me back if you have
any information.*

Thank you, Sarah

Reply from Dr. Surgical Oncologist:

Dear Sarah

The pathology report is available through the Mount Sinai Hospital which is probably why Dr. Medical Oncologist's office couldn't find it. The nodule that I removed was melanoma that had come back just under the skin in the soft tissues and I have been wanting to speak with you about the results and also about the MRI scan of the axilla which I reviewed again with the radiologist after we saw each other last. I know that my secretary was trying to get you to come in and see me. She offered you an appointment for last Friday. When she said that you did not want to come in I have been planning to call you to discuss the results but because of the long weekend I have not had the opportunity.

The problem is that I went around the nodule (what I could feel) but there were melanoma cells at the edges of what I took out. Also, the MRI suggests that there may be another nodule in the un-derarm....it looks worrisome and may be another recurrence in the soft tissue of the underarm. It seems to be in the lower underarm against the chest wall, not the upper part. I wanted to see you to re-examine you to see if I could identify it and also try and figure out what we should do next, first to try and see if it is true, try and find out where this is and what we should do about it. I would very much like to see you to re-examine you. Please let me know what you want me to do.

Secretary, can you please mail the pathology report from MSH [Mount Sinai Hospital] to Sarah? I excised an area from the un-derarm in June/July. Also please include her most recent MRI scan.

Dr. Surgical Oncologist

Me back:

WHAT?!

How could this information not have been relayed to me? I have been calling for a month. When I spoke with your secretary a couple of weeks ago, I asked her about the path and she said all she had was a note that I had my MRI and I needed to set up an ap-

pointment to have an excision. I said no, I already had the excision on the 25th. She said she'd look into it and then I never heard about it again. Obviously there was miscommunication, but how could it not have been sorted out sooner? I have called and left more messages. I should have just emailed you directly Dr. S.O. as this all got sorted out in a couple of hours.

So, I can see you ANY time and would like to see you, obviously, as soon as possible. I am completely shaken and in shock. Was not expecting this.

Thanks, Sarah

FUCK!!!!!!!!

posted by Sarah @ 11:12 PM   6 comments

APOLOGY ACCEPTED (BUT THAT DOESN'T MEAN I'M NOT PISSED)

From the secretary this morning:

Sarah,
The error is mine and I do apologize. The results I saw were
only from the earlier excision and not July 25th at Mt Sinai. I have
now found the results and faxed them to Dr Medical Onc's office.
As well, I have printed a copy of the MRI results and biopsy results
for you and may be picked up at the next appointment or could be
faxed or sent through regular mail.

An appointment is on hold for this Friday Sept 8th at 10:00
– this of course may be changed if not convenient for you. I will
leave a vm [voicemail message] on your home number regarding
this appt as well.

It is unfortunate that this lack of communication happened
and I will not make excuses on my part but will learn from this
experience.
Sincerely,

OK, mistakes happen. It was an unfortunate situation. She should have just asked the surgeon directly when she couldn't find the info I was looking for! I feel bad, because she's probably in deep shit now. She's new. I spoke with her this morning and she felt really bad. I was gracious without excusing her. I'm sure she has learned from this mistake. I'm sure her job is tough, juggling the scheduling of people who are sick and dying, dealing with them on the phone, fielding multiple demands from her surgeon and other doctors. I wouldn't want that job!

posted by Sarah @ 9:46 AM   4 comments

BORING DETAILS AND RANDOM TANGENTS

Blah. Bleh. Tired of this, but I can't be.

Edited to add: This entry ended up being very long and dry. It's for me so I have a record of my thoughts on all this. Seriously, unless you want to torture yourself, don't bother reading this entry! At least not in one sitting!

OK, so Friday. Friday, saw my surgeon. She apologized for telling me through email, but not for the delay. She says she was going to call me this week. Um, she should have called me a month ago. Whatever.

Turns out she (the surgeon) fucked up even more than that. This is kind of confusing so bear with me.

When I found that pea sized lump in my armpit in June, they did an MRI. The MRI confirmed a mass was present and the MRI report (which I finally saw for the first time on Friday, along with the path report from the excision) stated where the mass was located, and the size. The mass found on the MRI was about 2.5 cm round, as opposed to the small pea I was feeling and that my surgeon felt. Do you see where this is going?

Because we all felt a pea beneath my skin, my surgeon took that mass out. It was a recurrence. BUT, it was not the mass that showed on the MRI or the mass that was referred to in the MRI report. My surgeon took out what she felt, but obviously did not look closely enough at the MRI imaging or the report. If she had, she would have realized (and eventually did...) that there were in fact 2 masses that needed to be removed. One that was on the imaging, and one that was not (the pea). Just in case you are wondering, this mystery 2.5 cm mass is NOT the second mass that we were previously concerned about which turned out to be just scar tissue. Nope, I have a whole other tumour, have had it apparently for months, could have had it out in July, but there it is, still inside me. Neither of these showed on the CT scan (um, what are CTs good for exactly?) and only the larger one showed on the MRI. Crazy.

So, my surgeon admitted that mistake, but was not overly apologetic. I can sort of see it from her point of view. In her mind, this was a blunder, but the chances of it being a fatal blunder are very slim. A couple of extra months of this thing being in me is probably not going to make a difference in whether I live or die. It does make a difference to my sanity though. I know that sounds surprising to people reading who are not that familiar with certain aspects of advanced cancer. Certainly, it is better to get these tumours out than to leave them in, but statistically speaking, a couple of months delay in removing these suckers when they aren't in an organ or strangling an artery is unlikely to affect a person's overall survival. Statistically. On an individual level, of course it could theoretically make a difference. But, there is no way to ever know or to be able to measure that. Much the same way as, statistically speaking, my prognosis is shit. Take a 1000 people with stage 3C melanoma and they can tell you what percentage will be dead within 5 years and 10 years. It's not pretty. But they can never tell me that I won't be one of those people that will be alive in 10 years. Because there are some that are. There is no way of knowing what will happen to me. And that is why there is ALWAYS HOPE!

Anyfuckingway, what now?

I wait for another MRI date. I will harass the hospital on Monday and not wait for them to call me. It has been requested by my surgeon as "urgent". Based on past experience, that means the soonest I'll get the MRI is in 2 – 3 weeks. Backlog.

I will have another operation. This time (as with my first 2), I will be completely under and likely stay overnight in the hospital. I'll be sore. My arm is going to get fatter (lymphedema) and my range of motion will get even smaller. One day I should post pics of my armpit and pics of me trying to raise my arm over my head or put it behind my back. Ain't pretty. But, at least I still have use of it. I can still just reach my head to wash my hair! But I digress. Also based on past experience, my OR [operation] date will likely be in a 3.5 weeks to a month. That's the backlog for cancer surgery. Nothing new or surprising. It's the same for all cancer patients and has been the same in London and Toronto for me.

After that, there is talk of me entering a trial which I am mighty intrigued about and a bit miffed as it has not been mentioned to me before. I have to talk to my medical onc about this because it is possible that my surgeon is a bit confused. Usually, the trials start for my kind and stage of cancer in Canada when you hit stage 4 (distant mets or organ involvement) OR you have an unresectable (inoperable due to location/complications) local tumour. But so far I have had all resectable local recurrences. Knock on wood.

If I was in the U.S. there would be many trials that I qualify for and have qualified for. Not as much going on by way of research up here because we a) don't have the money, and b) don't have the patients. For those of you who have taken a statistics course, this makes sense, for those of you who are scratching their heads, just nod and smile. Makes more sense to wait for the results that come out of the trials in the U.S. for my stage and my cancer anyway.

Now, you're wondering why I don't go to the States for a trial. Trust me, I've thought about it and came to my decision back in January. It doesn't make sense for me to do that. It would cost me out of pocket for travel, consultations, blood work, scans, appts. with the U.S. doctors. In a trial, you are monitored very closely. They would want frequent scans and probably appts with me to check in possibly every week depending on the drug involved. I could maybe get my scans and bloodwork done here and send that stuff to the States so I didn't have to travel for those. But I would still have to pay for them because they would be above and beyond what OHIP (Ontario Health Insurance Plan a.k.a. Socialized Medicare for those of you outta province/outta country readers) is willing to pay for as part of my disease protocol. Factor in that there HAS NOT been a significant advance in the treatment of advanced melanoma in, well, ever, or 40 years or something. I'd be pretty dumb and naive to spend thousands and thousands of dollars to join a U.S. trial at this point. For me to actually hit on a trial that turns out to be the one is probably less likely than me winning the lottery next Friday. I'll save my money thank you.

My point was, before I struck another tangent, that I am very keen on this trial of which my surgeon speaketh. It would be free to me and I have nothing to lose. I don't know anything about it (yet!) except that if I do qualify (which I am sceptical about because of my stage 3 status and not stage 4) they will take part of my tumour, extract some lymphocytes [a type of white blood cell] which are the good "killer cells" and try to grow more. Then somehow or other through hocus pocus scientific stuff I don't understand (yet!) they will put all these lymphocytes back in my body and hope that gives my body the extra umph it needs to fight off the disease for good. Sounds interesting. Hey, it's something!

I'm also going to look at radiating the area again. This would be after I'm completely healed from the surgery. Last time, radiation wasn't recommended and I didn't want it again anyway. But I've been thinking about it more and talked with my surgeon about it and damnit all, we might just try it again.

My thinking is this towards radiating the local area:

Radiation in my disease does not increase overall survival statistically. What it does do is reduce the chance of recurrence in the local area by 80%. That's confusing. Basically what that means is, if you are fated to die this isn't gonna help you as the disease will just show up in another part of your body. But they can't predict who is fated and who isn't.

Now, I was radiated to my axilla (5 days/week for 6 weeks in Jan/Feb 2005) and this statistically should have meant that I would not recur in my axilla. I did though, BUT, even though the recurrence was still considered local, the tumour was about a centimetre OUTSIDE the field of radiation. Interesting. When the surgeon removed the tumour, she went through the same excision (scar by that point) from the removal of my first tumour and pulled the 2nd tumour through the area that was radiated and out of me. Then, I recurred in June back in the radiated area. Is it possible that as she was pulling the tumour out, cells broke off in the previously radiated area, once again infecting the area with melanoma? Yes, it is possible.

It is also possible (but admittedly unlikely) that because my body has now had 4 tumours appear in the same local area and nowhere else in my body, that my body is doing a fabulous job of not letting the disease spread elsewhere. MAYBE, just MAYBE there aren't any rogue cells travelling in by way of my blood and lymph fluid searching for that perfect place to set up shop and grow lethal tumours. MAYBE, just MAYBE all the bad cells are still local and have not travelled. So, I radiate the area AGAIN, this time a bigger area, and hope that it kills all the melanoma cells left behind and that none have already escaped to other parts of my body.

It just occurred to me that some people reading might be wondering why they can't just do some test to see if there are cancer cells in my body. There isn't such a test. I know, I always thought cancer would just show up in blood. Nope, imaging such as CT scans, X-rays, MRI can usually detect tumours depending on where they are and how big, but just because you don't have tumours doesn't mean you don't have microscopic cells floating around looking for a place to hide and form tumours. That's my layman's explanation and about the extent of my understanding of this crap.

That's why taking tumours out does not necessarily give a person the mythical "all clear". Depending on where the tumour was and other specifics of it, they can tell you what happened to a percentage of others in your same situation. Like with Sheryl Crow. She had stage 1 breast cancer in situ. It was caught very, very early because she was very, very lucky. Statistically, something like 95% of people in her exact situation won't recur and they gave her radiation just to be extra certain. She is really lucky if she is indeed in that 95% and because she likely will be, after a few years recurrence free, doctors will consider her cured if they don't already now.

Back to me and my radiation.... I have to have some serious chats with a couple of radiation oncs before the final decision is made. Radiation is never fun. It is going to be especially unfun to have it twice to the same area when the tissue will have an even harder time healing. I am still healing from nerve damage from last time which I won't even begin to describe except to say, holy

51

fucking bitch and ow. Radiating twice will mean more damage. And more lymphedema (fat arm!). Is it worth it? Statistically, not likely. Individually, maybe. Tough decision ahead.

Phew. That's it for now. Just wait for OR date, then figure out trial and radiation. This whole process (if radiation is going to be involved) will not likely be over until Christmas!!! At least I sort of know what to expect because I've been through it all before.

posted by Sarah @ 3:05 PM   4 comments

YOU SHOULD EAT MORE BLUEBERRIES

I know people mean well, but seriously...

If you know someone that is seriously ill, one of the worst things you can do is suggest books such as "You Can Heal Your Life" by Louise Hay, which ultimately just blame the patient for their problems OR tell them to eat more blueberries.

I don't care if you think I should eat more blueberries. All that tells me is that you are ignorant, and need to read something else other than Chatelaine [a Canadian women's] magazine.

Go eat more blueberries yourself. And while you're at it, think more positive, do yoga, go for Reiki treatments, spend $300 a month on supplements, get psychotherapy because obviously you don't love yourself, have more sex, carry crystals, don't drink from plastic, go to a clinic in Mexico, eat only organic or macrobiotic, start eating meat again, never have a drop of alcohol, meditate religiously, work out religiously, and think loving thoughts about everybody every second of every day. If you don't do everything I have suggested, then you obviously don't want to truly get better. And if you do do all these things and you still don't get better, it is because you didn't try hard enough or want it to work badly enough or you just plain didn't do it right.

After all, it is your fault.

posted by Sarah @ 3:46 PM   4 comments

CAMPING WITH DEREK

Derek and I drove straight from my appt. Friday in Toronto to Rock Point Provincial Park[11] on Lake Erie. It was beautiful! A bit rainy, a bit chilly at night, but we had a wonderful weekend. Had so much fun, just my boy and me!

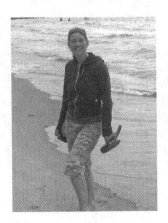
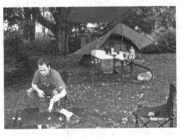

posted by Sarah @ 8:23 PM   1 comments

---

11 For information about Rock Point *www.ontarioparks.com/ENGLISH/ rock.html*

UNTITLED 1.0

Surgery is scheduled for October 2nd.

Here's an email to my surgeon I just sent which sums up my concerns at the moment.

morning

had mri on sunday. pretty sure i found yet another lump near scar line from my first two surgeries – bit bigger than a pea. also having constant pain in arm, hand, neck, upper back, little numbness in hand. T3s [Tylenol 3s] helping sort of. I can't help but think that there is something more than scar tissue going on elsewhere too as the whole area just seems to be getting harder and protruding more.

also, wondering if i will need to spend the night in hospital after surgery? i would definitely rather not unless absolutely necessary... first time i was fine going home, second i stayed in hospital but i think i would have been fine at home. it is your call, i'm not sure what the risks are to me leaving. i just know i'd be much more comfortable at home (sleep! and food!) and the expenses to my family in accommodation and food would be greatly reduced.

Thanks, sarah

   posted by Sarah @ 8:18 AM 0 comments

UNTITLED 2.0

Melanoma is out to get me. I just found another lump around the corner from my armpit sort of on my shoulder. Now, that's 3 I can feel. One on my side, lower armpit, and one right in my armpit by my old scar, and now this one. Holy shit.

I don't know what is going to happen, but I know this will not be fun.

I'm so sick of this. Why couldn't I have been one of the lucky ones?

Edited to add: I was going to delete what I just said because now that I am a bit more lucid I realize how ridiculous and self-pitying I am being and I'm rather embarrassed for myself. But then I figured, that was real in that moment. Just an example of the emotional swings. I had a bath and while I am totally heart-broken and terrified, my overwhelming mood right now is: Bring it on bitch! I'm taking you down!

posted by Sarah @ 12:42 PM   5 comments

NEW SURGEON REQUIRED

Sorry, to use copies of emails instead of actually blogging, but I'm too lazy to repeat stories which are already old and boring to me.

My surgeon has basically given up on me which I find appalling, maddening, frustrating, and illogical.

Her point is that since I've found more lumps (which by the way don't show up in the MRI done on Sunday – I ask again what the hell an MRI is good for if it can't even pick up tumours which are clearly larger than a pea!) the disease (statistically) will keep coming back therefore there is no point in removing them unless they cause me pain.

This is unacceptable to me at this point as I personally know of many who have only had local recurrences for years! And if I was at a major cancer centre in the U.S. they wouldn't hesitate to take these suckers out. Sure, chances are it will come back but a) it doesn't HAVE to as there are lucky people that deal with a bout like this and then something kicks in in their immune system and keeps the beast at bay for years, b) taking them out will at the very least slow down disease progression, c) it hasn't spread to organs yet so we must attack it where it is, d) um, every "treatment" offered once the disease has spread beyond the skin is not truly aimed at "cure" (because there is no cure) but in fact to "buy time" or slow down disease progression.

Maybe she has forgotten this or likes to believe that what she was doing up till this point was trying to cure me. Statistically, she wasn't going to cure me from the get-go. So why would she all of a sudden throw in the towel now? Delay progression. Keep it at bay until there is a cure. Keep it at bay for as long as possible. I'm fucking worth fighting for. I could be the exception to the rule and no one on my team should give up on me until I'm dead. I personally know of people with melanoma that spread to the brain that had it removed and are fine. This is soooo exceptionally rare, but you know what? This is my life and I have to believe that I could be that exceptional case too and my doctors need to do everything they can just in case I am that person. They don't know.

There is no doubt in my mind that if she was me, she would have the tumours resected. They are in the armpit for godsake and they are relatively easy to remove. Of course she would. Because it would buy her time, possibly. Apparently she had decided that I'm not worth the effort. But, because I'm a bitch, she's going to do it anyway.

Here's what transpired yesterday.

Surgeon:

If you are having more lumps, it is unlikely that local treatment such as surgery will be the best answer. It will only come back. MRI shows only one lump with some growth with local involvement of muscle but it is not seeing the small deposits. Local excision is only then used for the lumps that are symptomatic. I think that we should ask [Dr. Medical Onc] to reconsider systemic therapy....perhaps an experimental protocol? I think we should restage urgently with CT thorax/abdomen/pelvis to make sure everything remains localized. [Secretary] will call you with the appointment. It may be worth harvesting one of the lumps for that experimental protocol I was talking about but as far as I know we are still not using this for treatment. I will find out. For now we are keeping the OR date October 2 open for you regardless. I will be in touch.

My response:

I personally know of people going for years only experiencing local recurrences, and while I know what my odds are, I also know there certainly isn't any benefit to leaving these in. Taking them out could slow down disease progression... and since I'm already booked for the OR I especially don't see why they shouldn't come out. Also, something is causing my arm and hand enough pain that I am taking T3s around the clock and can't type or write without the meds. If systemic therapy is indicated then it would not be aimed at curing, but rather slowing down progression. Just the same, I don't see why the tumours that are resectable wouldn't come out, sure they might come back, but it may buy me more time. I could understand if I had organ involvement why you wouldn't bother with the axilla, but as far as we know (as of July) I do not. Knocking on wood that next CT confirms this. I'm not a statistic, and removing these masses could help me. If I were at MD Anderson[12], they would be resecting and resecting until it became unresectable. Just my two cents. Sarah

Surgeon:
That sounds like a plan. We will hold the OR time for you and do whatever we decide is right at the time.

It's fair to say I don't have much faith in my doctors right now. I wish I were in the States (if I were insured of course).

posted by Sarah @ 9:09 AM   2 comments

---

12 M.D. Anderson Cancer Center, Houston, Texas – a leader in cancer research and treatment. For information see *http://www.mdanderson.org/*

UNTITLED

Just me again. My surgeon (who is female by the way) just responded again to my email. This is the response I was looking for.

It just goes to show that you have to be your own best advocate with ANY doctor, do your own research, be on top of things, don't just roll over and accept what they say.

From my surgeon:

I understand your feelings and frustration. I am looking into options for aggressive surgical resection as well.

Now that's more like a team player. Sheesh man. Lucky I have the energy, education, language and confidence to fight these people a bit. What if English was my second language or I was too tired too fight or I was raised never to question authority. I am just steaming mad!

posted by Sarah @ 12:38 PM   2 comments

UNTITLED

Got another email from my surgeon. Seems my "team" has all banded together and I am to meet with them on Tuesday. That's me, Derek, Surgical Onc, Medical Onc (chemo doc), Radiation Onc, and probably more than one of each. I am to have a CT scan in the early afternoon to rule out further metastasis (spread), then we will hash out options and make some decisions as far as treatment. This is great news, usually they meet and talk about you when you aren't there. I've never heard of them all getting together at the same time with the patient.

I like that they keep using the word "aggressive" – as in "aggressive approach", "aggressive treatment", "aggressive surgical options". I think they got the point that I'm not playing the wait and see game. They say they are "extremely concerned" by the rate the disease is progressing in the radiated area. Ya, me too. It wasn't statistically supposed to recur there. Somewhere else yes, eventually, statistically, but not in the radiated area.

When I recurred outside the field of radiation in December '05, my surgeon, thinking she would do me a favour by using my old excision point and not create another nasty scar for me which would have been across my chest, re-entered the radiated area and dragged the new tumour back out through the old scar. It just makes so much sense to me that when she dragged it out, cells definitely would have broken off, re-infecting the radiated area. Also, that tumour barely had clear margins, I think it was less than a millimetre clear which is nothing. But what do I know? I was an English major, believe it or not. I didn't say I did well!

Anyway, it's plan time. Action time. I think they are going to re-stage me to stage 4. But I could be wrong there. Whatever, it's just a number anyway. A label. It doesn't change what my body is doing. What is, is. I mean, if the CT shows mets elsewhere then I am definitely stage 4. If not, then the staging is a bit murky. I'd post the staging charts, but I don't want to see them right now, as they always have survival stats attached to them. I know them by heart, but just seeing them in print or hearing them makes me shiver. I'm kinda at this weird borderline stage because the disease is definitely spreading, it just isn't spreading far. But it is spreading fast.

Oh, I found another lump today on the inside of my arm, about 3 inches from my armpit. It's deep, but I can feel it. So that makes the count I can feel up to....four.

I absolutely cannot believe I am at this point. My mind can't wrap around it. Will it ever? I don't know. The times I cope the best are when I can convince myself this isn't me I'm taking care of but someone else. I feel like there are two me's. The healthy me, and the cancer patient me. Hence, my life between Wonderland and Cancerland. I feel like the real me is the healthy me. I identify as healthy. I do not recognize this person who is supposedly sick. I can go through the motions and research, go to appointments and take treatments, but I don't feel like it is for me. I just can't believe this is me. It is the most bizarre feeling. A twilight zone. I suppose that is what is called dissociation, or is it disassociation? A coping mechanism. I don't want coping mechanisms, I don't want anything to have to cope with. But here I find myself.

Jeez, I just whine don't I? Poor me. I guess that's why this blog is good. No one hears this shit in real life. The thoughts just roll in my head 24/7, but no one hears it. I don't want anyone to hear it. I don't want others to feel my pain. I don't want to say my fear out loud because then it seems more real.

Derek has been buffering a meltdown every 1 – 3 months for the last 2 years. That was pretty good I think, considering. But since this last turn of events I've been having a meltdown daily. Except today, I think this rambling incoherence might be the equivalent of a meltdown though. What would I do without Derek? How is he so strong? It breaks my heart that I am breaking his heart. It breaks my heart that he has to worry, that he has to see me suffer. That he will see me suffer more.

OK, pity party done for tonight.

On a happy note, we tried out a new Japanese restaurant tonight for dinner and it was super delish! We both ordered the vegetarian bento box and it was the biggest bento I've ever seen with veggie maki, tempura (no egg in the batter, yay!), this mashed potato thing (Japanese?), miso soup, salad, veg gyoza, rice! What a feast. I ate the same amount as Derek, as per usual, no wonder I have a little pooch and a J-Lo butt. It's worth it to be able to eat well! I think eating is my favourite pastime.

I also finally got around to tidying up the office today. The desk has about 6 months of papers/bills piled on it waiting to be filed. It feels so much lighter in here now with those stacks not staring at me.

Oh, and the parking ticket I got outside Toronto General last Sunday was waived because apparently if you call to dispute, there is a one time waiver for first offences! I was all ready to dispute and took pictures of the street signs but had no idea how I was going to be able to fight a ticket in another city without spending more money on gas to get to court than the amount of the ticket. So, that was a pleasant surprise.

Well, it's late and I have to pee so I best say goodnight. Goodnight, sleep tight, don't let the bed bugs bite.

posted by Sarah @ 11:38 PM   6 comments

SEPTEMBER 28, 2006

OW

The pain in my arm is excruciating at times. It comes and goes, but mostly comes and stays. It hurts/aggravates to write/type so I won't be updating much until I've healed from surgery on Oct 3rd. It's the 3rd, not the 2nd. And who knows how long after that till my arm feels better.

I got bad news when I met with my docs the other day. They say there is tumour, behind all the scar tissue (what we were worried about in July!), that they can't take out. This was news to me because I have been told 3 times there was nothing there, but now all of a sudden there is? I am pissed, I don't understand. I have had my imaging sent to my London surgeon for a second opinion which I won't get till next week, after my surgery. Did I just confuse you?

My surgery Tuesday will be to remove the one tumour that is more on my side, kinda where your bra strap goes, so that they can keep it and maybe use cells from it in a vaccine trial that is set to begin at PMH in 6 months to a year. I am still fighting to have 2 other tumours removed as well (one sort of on my shoulder/back armpit, the other on my arm about 3 inches down from my armpit), as I know these are operable for sure. I am in so much pain. My arm bones ache, the skin on the back of my arm feels like it's on fire, my neck is kinked, my arm is useless. Pain meds are helping but not close to entirely. I got an oral morphine prescription today, and it is barely helping. This is all because these tumours are pressing on nerves or growing into nerves (hope not the latter).

I will be starting Interleukin-2 (IL-2) in a month or so which is a gruelling immunotherapy which will have me staying in a hospital in Buffalo for 5 nights, home for a week, then back to Buffalo for 5 nights and possibly this cycle will continue if the treatment seems to be working. My hand hurts too much and I'm too tired (and bored of this shit!) to talk more about it. It is going to suck, but there is about a 5% chance (yes, you read that right) that it could give me long lasting remission. There is a 15-25% chance it will give me short term remission. The reason I have to go to Buffalo is because although the drug is approved in Canada, they don't administer it. I don't want to get into the politics of why, but it looks like one day it will be available here, just not yet. In the meantime, the gov't pays for my treatment in the U.S. but my family has to pay for their hotel and food so they can be with me while I am in hospital.

How am I doing? Besides the pain, fine I think. I am in survival mode. I am living one day at a time, I do not think of the future... I am incapable of it, I think it is too painful. The mind does what it does, it makes things manageable. It's truly miraculous.

I feel like I got dealt some shitty cards here, but I also feel like my life is a miracle and I am in love with it. Now, I have to figure out if I mean that, or if that is the morphine talking.... I think I mean it. I am blessed. Whatever happens, I will be OK...

posted by Sarah @ 9:30 PM   6 comments

OCTOBER 02, 2006

PRE-OP

Going up to Toronto tonight for surgery tomorrow. Still have no idea what exactly they are taking out of me.

Went to Emergency last night because I couldn't take the pain. They gave me a shot of Toradol and a shot of Morphine then told me to double my prescribed dose of oral morphine. That did the trick. But holy crap, does this double dose ever make me sleepy! But it is nice to sleep well again after a week of not being able to get comfortable.

I don't imagine that I'll be able to update the blog for at least a few days after surgery because I don't think I'll have much use of my arm. I'll update as soon as I can.

This is a pic from 2 weeks ago. I think that was the last time I was out of my pyjamas. LOL[13].

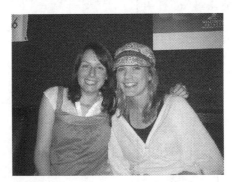

posted by Sarah @ 11:56 AM   9 comments

---

13 Cybercode for "laughing out loud"

HAPPY THANKSGIVING CANADA

I can't believe a week has passed since my last update. I have a lot to spew but I'm on heavy pain medication (methadone and gabapentin to be specific, and, no, I'm not a heroin junkie!) which has been keeping me sleeping for 15 hours straight, more if I let myself, and I usually do let myself. I have been walking around like a zombie, I'm so exhausted, seeing double, have no appetite, feel loopy but also a bit euphoric which is a bonus! And, I'm pretty much pain-free, however, I have major weakness in the arm and hand and loss of manual dexterity.

The reason I'm still having so much pain/nerve issues is because, as I expected, they didn't remove all the tumours. They only took out one which they are keeping to use for a vaccine trial that I may be able to partake in next year. So, the tumours that are in me, they press on nerves and that is where the pain comes from. So, sadly, this operation did not make me NED (no evidence of disease), but I knew that wasn't really the plan.

I didn't receive the second opinion from my London surgeon last week, but emailed him Friday and he said he would look at the imaging ASAP. I soooo hope to hear from him tomorrow, with some good news. I'm hoping he can make me NED!

I'll post more when I feel better. I need to get this medication adjusted because obviously I'm non-functional. I can't even drive... what am I saying? I can't even go for a walk I'm so plastered. I hope this all gets sorted out this week so I can live my life again.

posted by Sarah @ 6:37 PM   6 comments

HAPPY DANCE

I'm so happy!!!!!!!!!!!!!!!!!!

Just got off the phone with my London surgeon and he sees no reason why he can't resect all the tumours! Yes!!!!!!!!!!!!!!!!!!!

It may or may not make any difference to me long term, but he believes it is worth a shot! He is such a kind man, and is willing to do whatever he can to at least TRY and slow this disease down. At the very least, removing these tumours should get rid of my pain and restore strength and mobility to my hand if he doesn't inadvertently damage the nerves during surgery.

So, tomorrow I will get my OR date. I imagine it won't be for a month, but I can wait and I will be happy waiting.

IL-2 will have to wait till I'm completely healed and I suspect I won't even be a candidate for it once I am rendered NED by this surgery. The only way they can tell if IL-2 is working is by watching to see if tumours are shrinking. If I don't have any tumours to watch, then they don't know how much to give me. So, that's why I think chemo may have to wait. That's OK, most people who go on IL-2 have organ involvement so I'll save it for when/if that time ever comes!

This is the best news I've gotten in a long time!

You know what else is bizarre? My London surgeon says he sat down with the radiologist to look at the scans and she pointed out all the tumours. Toronto says they can only see one, the one that is "unresectable" and "don't know why" the other masses we can feel don't show on the scans. Whatever! They are idiots and don't know how to read scans!

Happy dancing I am!!!

posted by Sarah @ 4:27 PM 7 comments

LETTING GO OF DREAMS

My life. How it has changed.

I just noticed that my employer has posted the position that I was working towards before I got blind-sided by this stupid disease. Back in Sept 2004 I had just begun taking the final accounting course I needed to compete for this position at my workplace. Then, a couple of weeks later I was forced to drop out of the course due to my diagnosis and treatment. I was blissfully unaware of how much time I would in fact be off work, and in mid Oct 2004, a week after my first lymph node dissection, I competed for and won a competition for a job that was in direct line to me getting the position I really wanted, if only I got this course under my belt too.

I won the job, but I didn't start it until May 2006 after a year and a half of treatments and recovery. That's the good thing about working for the government and having a good union, they had to hold the position for me.

So, I started this job, one notch below the job I really want, in May 2006 and did it part time for 4 months up until this Sept when the other shoe dropped. I should add that in all my optimism, I had just re-enrolled for that course I need and got one week into it this time before having to drop out again, almost 2 years to the day that I first dropped out.

Now, I see in the newspaper that the position I had been wanting so bad, that I have taken courses for, that I have been groomed for, that I was envisioning as my "goal" is posted and it isn't going to be me filling it.

I have a hard time accepting that my life isn't actually going to go the way I had planned. I'm almost 30, just started my career, wanted babies, wanted grandbabies. Wanted to travel more, to experience more, to get to that point in your 40s that women say you just stop caring what other people think and fully accept and know yourself. I was playing soccer right up until the time I was diagnosed. I scored a goal the week before! I was fit, I was active, I was so on top of my game in all aspects of my life. We had just downsized to a small apartment from a 3 bedroom house we were renting to save money for a down payment. I was doing well in my part-time studies and getting praise at work. I was feeling so confident, sharp, on top of the world. I knew that even though there were setbacks here and there, that things would always be OK.

Someone else is going to take my job. Everyone else gets to lead the life I wanted to live. I know that's not true, but in my daily life it is. I'm the sick one. I'm that girl who people lower their voices to talk about and say, "It's such a shame, I feel so bad for her". I don't want to be a tragic story. It isn't supposed to be my story! I know my story and for fuck sakes, I know this isn't it!

I'm at a loss. I'm so sad. I don't know what to do. I know I have to "fight", but this is a war I didn't wage and don't believe in. I'm no warrior, I'm just a normal girl who had a normal life and as the months go on and the setbacks get closer together, I feel like I am watching my normal life disappear more and more.

This last month has been hard because it has been entirely about cancer. I have officially moved from Wonderland, to a limbo between Wonderland and Cancerland, to living full-time in Cancerland. Where before, my cancer life was just one small slice of a full pie… I was back at work, I was jogging, I was going out to pubs, concerts, camping, trips to New York and London [England], starting school… now I do nothing but sit around in a methadone haze, make phone calls and visits to cancer doctors, watch TV, surf the net, read and think. Think think think. Try to solve this unsolvable problem. My mind just goes in circles, trying to figure out the answer to this riddle: How do I get better and stay better?

I just hope this surgery will indeed alleviate the pain so I can be off the methadone, and get out and about more after I've healed from surgery. Even if I'm not at work, I feel like a fuller human when I can at least feel good and pretend I'm just on vacation. I can easily pass my time when I feel good, go window shopping, coffees at Chapters, yard work, house work, meeting people for lunch, maybe hopping on the elliptical trainer we bought 2 weeks before I got the news of this latest recurrence. It sits in the living room, a constant reminder of how good I felt only one month ago. A constant reminder that my best intentions were yet again squashed, that hoping and having goals and dreams does not mean they will actually come true.

It gets really painful to keep "moving forward" when your dreams keep getting squashed like that. It is so demoralizing to have to keep picking myself up and brushing myself off and try-ing again.

The first time this happened was when I won that job competi-tion and realized that I wasn't actually going to be able to start it for a long time.

The second time was in Dec 2005. I had just finished my inter-feron treatments, was looking forward to returning to work in the new year and bought myself a whole new wardrobe of work attire. Two weeks later I found a lump. I wasn't going to be going back to work for a while. I had to return all my clothes knowing the soonest I'd be at work was the spring, so no point in having a new winter wardrobe. Returning those clothes was one of the hardest things I've ever done because of what they symbolized. They sym-bolized my optimism, my hopes for the future, me getting my life back after over a year of it being high-jacked by surgery, radiation and interferon treatments.

The third time was in late June when I found that little lump. I had gotten myself to the point physically where I was jogging 5k for the first time in my life (I'd always been relatively active with soccer, gym, ex-swim instructor, but never been able to run outside straight for half an hour). Even though it wasn't logical, I had somehow hoped that being that physically fit would keep the cancer away. The fear was always there, because I know it doesn't work that way, but I just hoped so badly that the universe would see how badly I wanted to stay healthy and how much I appreciated my body. I was looking for divine justice, a divine intervention, but I know there is no such thing.

The fourth time was just over a month ago, when I was forced to really admit for the first time that this "problem", my cancer problem, is huge. I am caught in a one step forward, two steps back cycle that is likely to continue this way, despite my greatest hope and wish. I am a full-time cancer patient right now. Trying hard not to let it define me, but really, I don't have much of a life outside cancer pain, cancer treatments, medicine and appointments right now. Cancer has been my full-time job for the last month. It's getting old and I'm so over it. So bored of this story, I keep saying that. I'm so bored of it.

Everything happens for a reason, what doesn't kill us makes us stronger, things always work out in the end, and if they don't, we find a reason why it was "for the better anyway". These are the mantras we all tell ourselves so we keep on keepin' on through thick and thin. Those mantras don't cut it for me anymore unfortunately. Forced out of blind naiveté, my mantras today are:

We are only guaranteed this moment, so make the most of it.

Shut up and stop wallowing as it is ruining your experience of today.

Take comfort in the fact that others have been down this road before you, you can do it too.

Death is only a continuation of life.

There is no such thing as death.

Hopes and dreams are just an illusion; all we have is the present.

I have to explain that last one in my next post. There is a story that goes along with it, making them the most comforting words that I have heard since the beginning of this journey. I repeat it all the time, because of the way it came to me, and because of how true it is.

posted by Sarah @ 7:34 PM   6 comments

TAKE THIS OPRAH!

I always knew I was meant to be a mother. OK, not always, but since my early 20s. Since that time in most peoples' lives that they begin to question their place in the world, what they will contribute to this planet, their raison d'être.

When I was searching for my purpose, for what I wanted to do with my life and how I could better the planet, I found myself frustrated by the fact I had no desire to contribute to a "cause". No desire to be an environmental activist or advocate for the poor. I've never been overly concerned with those macro issues, interested, but not concerned enough to really get involved in anything like that on a large scale. I never wanted to save the world and I felt guilty about that.

A deep longing to be a mother overcame me during that time (and still now, although I am trying hard to let it go), a desire so deep that I literally ached in my uterus sometimes and had to preach at myself to use protection because I hadn't finished school or started my career. I would (and shamefully/painfully still do when I'm weak) walk through baby departments in stores and pick out in my mind clothes, furniture, accessories for my future child. I'd watch those birth story shows on reality TV and fantasize that it was me. I knew my time would come.

After some time and reflection, I realized that I was put on this earth to be a mother. My purpose was not to affect change on this planet on any kind of macro level; it was to love and raise another human being, pure and simple. Perhaps to love and raise a human being that would go on to make bigger changes in the world. But for me, I just knew my job was at home. In this life, I was to be a kind, decent, and caring person in my day-to-day life, and affect just the people around me in a better way. If we all could just commit to being kind in our daily lives, then there would be no war. That was my commitment to the world, and my purpose was to raise another human being who would learn the same compassion and pass it on.

This was a spiritual realization. I believed in my path, almost like it came to me from God, the Universe, whatever you want to call it. I also believed, on this same level, that I would have a long life, sure there would be pain and suffering, and there was, but I just knew I was meant to live a long full life, raise children, and make the world a better place by being a good, compassionate person in my daily life.

So now, I question my every thought and belief. What is the point in pursuing spirituality or faith when the messages I believed came from a higher source turned out to be mere fabrications of my mind. Or perhaps this was to be my path, but things such as cancer and illness are out of the scope of God's control? A physiological accident happened, it was discovered at too late a stage for treatment to be effective, and now my path has changed?

There is no point in searching for meaning in all this because I can't trust the meaning I find. Gah! I don't know what my point is. Nothing too brilliant. I guess I'm just having a pity party and whining that life isn't fair. Why do people who don't even want kids get accidentally pregnant, or people who are ambivalent but just have babies because they want someone to take care of them when they're old, while women who really want kids suffer from infertility or illness? I guess I just want to scream: Yes, bad things happen to good people! Good things happen to bad people! There is such a thing as being lucky and unlucky, and a lot of what happens in this life is absolutely random! Take that Oprah!

I'm just so tired of feeling like this is my fault or people implying that I can change it with visualization or positive thinking. Let me see you cure your next cold with positive thinking, and let me see you cure your next bout of food poisoning by visualizing an army of white blood cells attacking the bacteria! That would never occur to these people, but somehow they think that cancer is different? Ya, it's different, it is a hell of a lot more serious, powerful, sneaky and deadly! It is also incurable at late stages.

Most people that are cured were lucky enough to have the cancer discovered at an early stage. Plain and simple. There are 4 stages of cancer, each stage tells you how far the cancer has spread from the primary location. 90% of breast cancer patients are cured. Same with melanoma. That is because almost 90% get the cancer cut out surgically at stage 1 or 2. They had some sign of the cancer early on in the disease and got it removed before it spread. The people that die are almost all (there are exceptions to the rule) comprised of people who were unfortunate in that their disease wasn't discovered early because there were no symptoms, or they were misdiagnosed, or they ignored the symptoms until stage 3 or 4.

When you find out if someone has cancer, find out what stage they are to know how serious it is and how likely they are to survive. All cancer diagnoses are not equal, as our media would have us believe. A lot of the "warriors" and "survivors" that we see on TV, I've mentioned Sheryl Crow before, we are led to believe survived because of sheer determination, positivity and strength of character. Nope, I dare say, they survived because they had itty bitty cancers in situ[14] that have less than a 10% chance of spreading! Then they sometimes go through radiation or chemo on top of surgery just to make sure that the cancer doesn't come back.

Sure, the treatment sucks and they were scared, and lives changed forever. But the media makes them out to be these rays of hope and living testaments to the power of will and determination, when in fact, they were just damn lucky. The media perpetuates the myth that cancer can be beaten with positive thinking and by not presenting us with the facts of the disease.

Lance Armstrong. Here is a lucky guy. Sure, his testicular cancer spread to his lungs and brain making him a stage 4 cancer patient, but wouldn't ya know it, Lance Armstrong happened to get one of the few cancers that are curable at stage 4! Even with metastases to the brain, our beloved Lance STILL had a 50% chance

---

14 In situ normally means "in the natural or original position or place"; however, Sarah's meaning is "in a confined area".

of surviving long term! Lance was lucky that only a few years before his diagnosis an effective chemotherapy agent was discovered to cure many cases of advanced testicular cancer! When breast or melanoma cancers spread to the brain one has less than a 5% chance of surviving five years because there is no cure for stage 4 of these diseases. What Lance had to go through to get cured was horrifying, but it was no miracle that he survived. And it wasn't because he was some kind of super human, a pillar of strength and determination. It wasn't because, as he says, he just refused to die. It was because he called heads and that's where the coin landed.

He had a 50-50 shot at his very worst. My cancer hasn't spread to any organs and I have way less than a 50-50 shot at survival because there are no effective treatments yet. Lance Armstrong didn't survive because he is a good person, a strong person or because he wanted to live more than anyone else does. His got dealt a good last hand.

Dana Reeve died of lung cancer, only months after she was diagnosed, as most lung cancer patients do, because symptoms do not present until a later stage, when it is incurable. Some suggested that she unconsciously just wanted to be with her late husband, Christopher Reeve, or that she brought it on herself by not taking care of herself while tending to Chris for all those years. The cancer myth in reverse. The truth is that Dana, from all outward appearances, was full of light, life, and positivity. She exuded peace, happiness, and strength in any interview I ever saw with her. She was unlucky that cancer developed in her, and doubly unlucky that she got a cancer that had a bad prognosis from the beginning. Simple as that. Life is not always fair; bad things happen to good people for no reason that we can understand.

I'm just going with the flow. What will be, will be. I think that is a totally OK way to go about coping with this illness. I hope for the best, but I am realistic. We hear those stories of survivors who beat all odds, and attribute it to something they did or thought, when we have no idea why they made it and no doctor would claim to know. For every person that was "healed" by a healer or some herbal concoction, there are thousands more that healed spontaneously on their own. Because it does happen. Most people who survive advanced cancer don't do anything special. And most people that do do something special or extreme die. That's the truth, reality. I live in reality and I'm sick and tired of ignorant misinformed but well-meaning people offering their misguided advice because if I reject it, they conclude in their minds that I just don't care about myself enough to "fight". Bullshit.

A recurring thought popped in my head today while I was getting marked by ultrasound for my upcoming surgery (oh, I haven't mentioned yet that my surgery to remove hopefully all the tumours is this Thursday, Oct 19th!). This whole process from beginning to now, and I imagine forward, has just been so damn interesting! Yes, quite horrifying, but I am always just so interested in how things play out, how things get done, the machines, the doctors, the process, the research. I wouldn't wish this on anyone, but since it is me, I can often sort of step outside myself and watch what is unfolding as if it were a television docu-drama. Cancer, cancer treatment and support, and the emotional side of cancer (which I read a lot about) are fascinating subjects that I was 100% blind to before it became my reality. Through all the fear and pain and disfigurement, I am morbidly entertained by this whole process at times. Not in a funny "ha ha" sort of way, just in an awe inspired "that's neat!" kind of way. I suppose a psychologist would call that a coping mechanism. I'm a fan of coping mechanisms.

Ya, so my surgery is on Thursday. Apparently I'm not staying the night, but I'll really be surprised if I don't. If he actually does cut it all out, I'm going to have gashes in 2 places on my arm, my whole right armpit will be gutted and a huge area on my shoulder will be excised where there are 2 tumours. I'll definitely post pics. I'm going to have Frankenarm! Hey, that's the least of my worries. Well, come summer I'll be crying about it because I can't cover up the scars and my fat arm, but for the winter I'll pretty much be able to forget about it once the wounds heal.

As for IL-2 in Buffalo, it is a no go. If the tumours all come out, I can't have the chemo as I suspected. My onc in Toronto said "It'll just come back" when I told him I was having surgery here in London. I said, I know it probably will but we'll deal with it then. Seems logical to me to take it out, bang up my arm but give me some cancer free time. If it comes back, well, I'll just do IL-2 then. It's not like the chemo is a proven cure or anything, so why jump on it and be sick and miserable for weeks when I don't have to? And if IL-2 doesn't work, then that will just lead into me trying every other chemo available which will make me sick for months and months. Why go down that road right now? I'd rather get cut up thank you.

Well, I guess I'll update after I get cut up, unless I feel inspired tomorrow. I still want to write about "hopes and dreams are just an illusion".... another time though.

posted by Sarah @ 12:16 PM   11 comments

TWILIGHT ZONE

My surgery in London was a great success by all accounts. My dear London surgeon – who you just have to like, he is so jovial and genuinely caring – reported to my parents and Derek in the waiting room right after the surgery that they got everything out and that it was no problem.

He had no idea why Toronto wouldn't take them out, especially in someone young and otherwise healthy like me. We were happy, I was happy. Even though I knew that my journey with melanoma was statistically likely not over, I just felt lighter knowing it was all out and that there was always hope it wouldn't come back. I was discharged from the hospital that day, and back at home helping (a teeny bit) with supper that evening. Besides some arm pain, I felt surprisingly good. Anaesthetics and Percocets don't seem to affect me like other people.

Friday afternoon, the day after the surgery, a home care nurse came to visit, empty my drain [used to insure that the surgical site does not collect the extra fluid the body normally produces after an operation], and change my bandages. I took the bandage-free opportunity to poke around and was stunned to find a lump, about the size of a dried apricot, right in the area that was supposedly gutted – sorta between my armpit and boob. OK, really, I wasn't stunned. I was not surprised at all. It was more kinda like, "Of course this is happening. Mistakes always happen with me. This sucks." I didn't freak out, I called the surgeon's secretary to see if I could get a clinic appointment with the surgeon on Monday. She didn't call me back, but in her defence, I called only a half hour before she left for the day.

First thing today (Monday morning) I called again. The secretary answered and got me in for 10 am when I explained what happened. When I met with the surgeon, he first said, oh, it must be a seroma [a pocket of clear benign fluid that sometimes develops in the body after surgery]. But then when he felt the mass I could see he was confused and concerned. He babbled about how he couldn't believe they could have missed anything. They marked that whole area, they dug in that area...

He took out a syringe to see if he could drain fluid, hoping it was a seroma or cyst... something other than melanoma. The syringe didn't draw any fluid. Oh, oh. Possibly big boo boo. I can't be mad at this guy because he is just so nice and personable and I really really like him! And he just seems to care so much about me. He is booking me for an ultrasound to determine what this is, and if it is a missed tumour I'll be in for surgery again and he will feel like a big incompetent goof.

I know mistakes happen but geez, I'm tired of them happening to me. There are many more that have happened in this two year journey – things that are just plain crazy which I haven't talked about here as this blog only began in May. It is surreal to think this mistake could have happened as they had the surgeon, residents, an ultra sound technician and a radiologist... this was an ultrasound guided operation and they went over my whole arm, back, chest, axilla with the ultrasound looking for tumours. And this mass is literally millimetres from where they excised! He didn't deny that it was possible, but seemed very mystified as to how. He said "bigger mistakes have happened, as you know, because they keep happening to you. This really sucks."

He's right. It does really suck. It sucks so much that I feel like I'm in an alternate reality. I feel like I've entered the twilight zone.

Standby.

posted by Sarah @ 12:47 AM   5 comments

OCTOBER 24, 2006

I COMPLAIN TOO MUCH

Thanks for standing by.

Ultrasound today. Confirmed tooma. They missed one! Right in the area they gutted. Good lord. Scheduled for another surgery on Nov 3rd. That's 4 surgeries in exactly 1 month. Big oops. Who do I trust? Why is everyone so incompetent? I feel like I just complain and complain, but it's not me, right? Everyone else seems to be fucking up.

Here's the list of fuck-ups:

1996: Mole from my back removed and biopsied. Removed because I didn't like it, aesthetically. Pathology report said it was an atypical spitz nevus, which is a benign kind of mole. As you can see from the article I linked to below[15], this kind of benign mole is often actually melanoma, misdiagnosed. I had no idea at the time (I was 18) and I went on merrily with my life for 9 years before I found that egg size lump in my armpit in Sept 2004. Which by the way was the size of a softball by the time it was surgically removed a month later. I do feel lucky I got 9 years till my recurrence though... this is unusual as most people will recur within 2 years.

Geez, how that would have changed my life if I recurred at 20. Because in those 9 years, I got a degree, I experienced living in Toronto for 5 years, I met some amazing people and made some good friends, I met Derek, I backpacked [with him] in Mexico

---

15 http://www.ncbi.nlm.nih.gov/pubmed/15249862?dopt=Abstract

(twice) and Guatemala, I got a decent job with the Ontario government for 3 years which led to a better job/career with the Ontario government which I just began as I talked about in a previous post. I grew up. But I digress...

Nov 2004 – Dec 2005: Adjuvant therapy interferon. I was not told that I had any other option than this drug (many doctors offer the option of doing nothing as interferon is a controversial treatment option).

I should have been told of the controversy over interferon. I should have been told that I would feel like crap for a year in exchange for an average recurrence free time of 12 months in people who are destined to recur. I was high risk for recurrence, but many people who are high risk don't recur whether or not they do this treatment. If you are going to recur, you will at some point but no one can predict who will and who won't. This I learned on my own, well into my treatment.

Apparently, the latest study shows that interferon helps approximately 9% of patients stay recurrence free. That was not the information available at the time I started. Anyway, knowing that now, I would have chosen interferon anyway for that 9% chance. But, apparently I wasn't one of those 9% anyway. Cancer Care Ontario has a protocol for administering this drug and it states that oncs should talk to their patients about the pros and cons of this drug so they can decide for themselves if it is something they want to do. I was never given that option.

Dec 2005: Maybe I wasn't one of those 9% because the whole 10 months I was injecting myself with interferon, I was on the wrong dose! I was on a lower dose than I should have been and I only found out 8 months into the treatment because I found on the internet the formula they use to calculate the dosage and realized mine was wrong!

By that time, I had switched medical oncologists. He said he has no idea why my previous onc would have prescribed me a lower dose but since I was almost done the treatment and there was no research/study to suggest that a lower dose wouldn't work, that I might as well just continue with the lower dose. You would think that the pharmacist or my new onc would have realized my dose was wrong. And if my old onc did it on purpose (which I think he did because I questioned him about it via email at his new job in Miami and his rationale was stupid and senseless!). He should have told me he wasn't giving me the full dose, at which point I would have questioned it. A patient should be informed of these decisions, dontcha think?

Dec 2004: I was in the chemo suite, hooked up to my IV [intravenous] drip of high-dose interferon (I did this every weekday for a month before I started the 10 months of self injection at home) but waiting for my nurse to start the drip. Another nurse (luckily) walked by, looked at the bag hooked up to my IV, looked at me, and whispered to my nurse that it wasn't my name on the bag and rolled her eyes at her. My nurse swiftly unhooked that bag and replaced it with a bag that had my name on it. I was this close (holding thumb and index finger an inch apart) to being administered someone else's chemo drug! How does that happen?!!!!! Very frightening, who knows what would have happened to me.

That I believe was the last fuck-up before the shenanigans of this past summer and fall started. When you tally it all up, it seems rather unbelievable. It gets frustrating, especially when it's different doctors and nurses. I am just feeling like I can't trust anything anyone says or does, when I always held doctors on a pedestal. Nope, they are just human, and they make mistakes like everyone else. But, the difference is when they make mistakes, they are dealing with peoples' lives.

But, alas, I can't complain too much, because at least they are trying and at least I am getting some care. Millions of people around the world don't get any care for their diseases, yet my government is spending thousands and thousands of dollars on me, on a disease that they know is incurable at this point... but they try anyway! They try to buy time for me until there is a cure. Literally, they are buying time. Thank you Canadian tax payers!!!!

My interferon alone cost about $30,000 Canadian, if I ever do end up going to Buffalo for IL-2, this treatment costs the government $250,000 for only a 5% chance it will give me a long remission. Not to mention the hundreds of free doctor visits, scans, ultrasounds, blood tests etc etc etc. For this, I have to feel blessed. People die everyday in pain and agony because there are no treatments like mine, there are no pain medications, and if there are they certainly can't afford them in third world countries. I can't forget this. When I complain, I must remember how really lucky I am. Gosh, for so many reasons, I really am very very lucky. And most of you reading this are too. Don't forget that and don't take what you have for granted.

posted by Sarah @ 10:45 AM   4 comments

CRACKED OUT

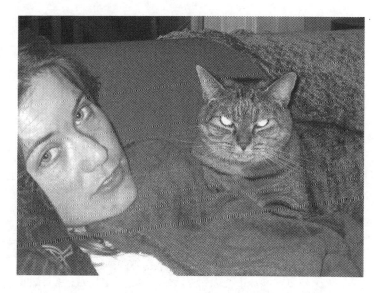

Me [and Misty] a couple of weeks ago when I was blasted from too many pain narcotics. Those eyes say it all. Luckily we've got the medication figured out for the most part (still in pain sometimes though) so I don't look like a total junkie anymore!

posted by Sarah @ 4:12 PM   1 comments

INSPIRATION AND HOPE

Karen Velasquez is a member of MPIP [Melanoma Patient's Information Page] and gives all us melanoma warriors hope. She was diagnosed stage 4 ten years ago today! Beating the statistics to the ground. While she isn't NED, somehow her tumours have been kept in check by treatments and her body, and have not been fatal. Karen has been an outspoken melanoma activist, warning people of the dangers of the sun and to be aware of any changes on their skin. She even appeared this year on the Dr. Phil show to warn people about the dangers of tanning beds. She is a true inspiration.

Here is some of her history in her own words taken from her MPIP Patnet[16]:

I was dx [diagnosed] in 1992 with the primary mole on my back, clarks level 3. I had WLE (wide local excision) and was told everything was OK. In Oct of 1996, I was dx stage 4 with mets to my jawbone, lymph system (32 tumors) and spots on my liver. I was treated at The National Cancer institute with high dose IL2 with GP100 Vaccine as well as the Flowpox vaccine. I did nine rounds of IL2/vaccine combo and all the disease went away with the exception of the jawbone, I had my jaw removed and reconstructed. My NED time lasted 2 years. Since that time I have not had any other chemical treatment, but have had 4 additional surgeries for lymph tumors, and had radiation to a bone marrow met to my left femur. This disease seems to have become more of a chronic disease rather

---

16 To read more, go to *http://www.mpip.org/library/pperspective.html*

than a fatal one for me. The IL2/vaccine combo seems to have slowed things down. I am scanned every three months for follow up. I believe that this is the key to maintaining long term survival. Without that constant monitoring, these tumors would likely have become a bigger issue.

Another inspirational person everyone in cyberspace should meet is Heather[17]. Heather has not posted on her blog in 2 weeks and I, as well as everyone at MPIP, am very concerned. I'm not a prayer (prayerer? huh?) but I do hope she is OK. I'm so worried. Heather, if you are reading this, we are all thinking of you!!

I have surgery on Thursday to remove the tumour my surgeon missed. Just as well he missed it because I just found 2 more curious lumps on my upper arm. Damn. Hopefully he'll take those out too. It just comes out of nowhere. I can't believe how fast my tumours grow. Whatever.

On a brighter note, my pain seems to be under pretty good control with the Methadone and Percocets and my mood is good too, besides the frustration and anger towards the medical community right now.

And, on an even brighter note, my beautiful fur-babies Misty (brown) and Mojo (B&W) make me smile and warm my heart every time they are near (except when they scratch the couch or whine for food before the alarm goes off in the morning!)

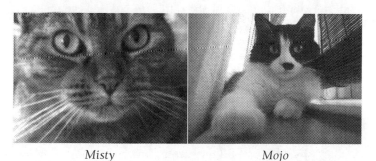

Misty   Mojo

posted by Sarah @ 5:29 PM   8 comments

---

17 www.livingwithmelanoma.blogspot.com

MAKEOVERS ARE FUNNER THAN SURGERIES! WHO KNEW?

Had surgery on Nov 2 to remove 5 masses. I know 4 are melanoma, the 5th is a little lump I found in my right breast a couple of days before the surgery. Waiting for path results.

As of Sunday, Oct 29th, I have lost mobility in my right wrist, elbow, and most of my fingers. I scribble like a 5 year old when I sign my name. I am typing with my left hand and right index finger only. I have been wearing a hat because I can't manipulate my hands to use a hair elastic and I don't have enough arm strength to blow dry my hair. I'm getting used to it though and finding other ways to do things. In the pics, no hat because I had friends to do my hair!

My surgeon is concerned about this, so I stayed the night in hospital because they said that way I'd be first in line for MRIs and CTs if spots came up. And they did. I had 2 CTs and an MRI. I know my brain is clear of mets which is a huge relief, because loss like this can be a sign of cancer spread to the brain. It is more likely that there is a tumour growing in or near the brachial plexus nerves but I'll get an answer to that next Friday. It could just be scar tissue infringing on the area from the Oct 19th surgery – that's my theory and hope! Geez, it hurts to type. My blogs might be short and sweet for a bit till they get my hand working again!

Went out last night for a friend's early birthday and had lots of fun. No drinkin' though since I'm popping Methadone, Percocets and Gabapentin! We had our faces done at MAC Cosmetics then went out for Thai. Lookin' pretty hot 48 hours after cancer surgery if I do say so myself!

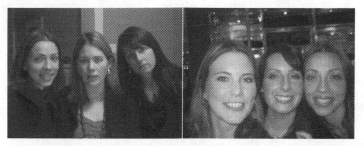

Pre-makeover. No make up.
Trying to look pathetic.

Post-makeover! Hot chicks!

posted by Sarah @ 8:58 PM   5 comments

PERI-OPERATIVE NURSING INCIDENT

I'm going back in time for this entry to over two weeks ago following my Oct 19th surgery. I want to say that my most recent surgery on Nov 2nd was a relatively peaceful experience, filled with lovely nurses and staff who made me feel like a person, who made me feel cared for and who I was able to trust.

On Oct 19th, however, even though it was the same hospital, I had a bunch of snarky, bitter, angry nurses who I can only assume are counting down the days to retirement, because they obviously no longer love what they do and sadly probably have had too many years of feeling underappreciated, undervalued and stretched too thin.

Let me preface this by saying I fully realize this is possibly the least professional email I have ever written in my life. I don't even think I read it over as it was an utter chore to do, when I just wanted to let the incident go. This email is to the "Manager, Perioperative Care" at her request following a show-down I had (who me? can you believe it?) with one of her nurses immediately following my Oct 19th surgery.

The manager was a lovely woman who completely understood my point of view (or so she made me think?) and was evidently highly adept at conflict resolution. This "letter" was a bullshit piece of red-tape that she required for her follow-up with the nurse, presumably to help assess if any disciplinary action was required. She needed something in my writing, even though we rehashed the event through my tears while I lay in my hospital bed ad nauseam.

She knows the story, I was post-op and couldn't write, type, think, or care less about re-visiting this incident so this is what I sent off for "the file". It may not make sense to anyone else but her and me, but I am posting it for myself, because it is what happened to me. It is a piece of my story and shows how frustrated I can get in my cancer journey when forced to deal with people who have no common sense or respect for basic human dignity.

hi,

sorry i have not written to you about the bathroom fiasco. honestly, i have been in too much pain and also have no use of my right hand so it has been at the back of my mind. i just want to forget it. forgive me, but i will just quickly write out what happened in this email instead of a formal letter. you can print it.

i appreciate that the nurse came to apologize and i accepted it after it was modified. she was stuck on the "i thought you were dizzy" excuse and i "didn't hear you say you were OK the second time" which didn't explain why she proceeded to break in the bathroom while I was screaming "what the hell are you doing, and get out!". she only left when i yelled at her more and got off the toilet to motion her out. i said i'd keep the door unlocked after that if she stood right there (anyone could have come in) but after a few minutes (i still couldn't pee) i got up to check if she was there and she wasn't. when she walked by that's when i proceeded to yell at her in front of everyone saying she had no right to come in the bathroom when a patient says they are fine, that she had no respect for patient dignity, crossed the line, and was very rude. she denied all this which just infuriated me more. i went back in the bathroom and locked the door and cried because i always feel like a "bad patient" for standing up for myself.

my feeling is that if she absolutely thought there was something wrong (makes no sense why she would after i said twice thru the door i was fine), a respectful nurse who thinks of her patients as human beings deserving of respect and as much dignity as possible considering the setting, would explain thru the door why she was worried and felt she had to check on me, then open the door slightly to peep in. once she saw that i was sitting calmly on the toilet, she should promptly leave after apologizing for the intrusion. that i could have handled.

instead, this woman busted in with no warning, just saying, "I'm coming in!", as I yelled no! She walked right in and refused to leave until I actually had to yell at her and then get up off the toilet! Completely senseless. What, did she expect me to pee while she stood beside me? I had 100% come out of the anesthetic like I always do. Sure, it was right after I came out of recovery, but I was in recovery for 1/2 hour and sitting up, talking and asking for magazines within 10 minutes post-op. I walked to the bathroom myself and told her twice I was fine. She was WAY out of line and I've never been so shocked in my life – her behaviour was so bizarre.

i immediately thought she was thinking i was shooting up heroin in the bathroom. i told her i was on methadone, asked to get my bag to change in to my pants before going to the bathroom. when i was in the bathroom for so long and couldn't pee (a side effect of methadone) i think she decided i had gotten my supplies out of my bag and was shooting up. many nurses have immediately thought i was a junkie when they heard i was on methadone. they never ask why or if they do they don't believe me because it is so rare. now i have a letter to carry around with me. my methadone is for severe cancer pain and is prescribed by dr. F. this is the only thing i can think of that would warrant such bizarre behaviour from a nurse.

her apology was weak at first because she stuck to the dizzy excuse which makes no sense as i've already explained. when i told her that i thought she had lost sight of the fact that her patients are people first who deserve to be treated how she would want to be treated, i think she better understood my complaint and i accepted her apology when she said she had learned a lesson and would never do that to anyone again.

thanks for your patience and understanding when we met. i will be having more surgery this thursday and hope not to run into anything like this.

sarah

What can I say, I'm a hot head sometimes! I have zero tolerance for people disrespecting me and I don't always handle these situations myself in a dignified way. I'm a yeller, and a screamer, and if that doesn't work I become a crier. Something to work on I guess. Excuse me while I bow my head in shame. I am almost 30, right? But in my defence, that nurse was clearly over the line!

posted by Sarah @ 1:40 PM   4 comments

JUST KEEP CHOPPING AND IT'LL ALL BE BETTER TOMORROW

Right.

So, the swelling and bandages are gone from my Oct 3rd surgery with the bat [surgeon] in Toronto that "couldn't" or more likely didn't want to treat me further. There is a pretty little scar, and I was just poking around and what do I feel? A lump! Right under the scar, the same size as what she supposedly took out. So, am I to think it grew out of nowhere or did she just take a bit of it out (see blog entries late Sept/early Oct 2006 for background) instead of the whole thing?

And if so, why did my new surgeon not see it, even though I JUST had surgery about 2 cm away from the site only 4 days ago? Even though I've had supposed ultrasounds to the area and been poked and prodded. Whatever! Oh, did I mention: Cancer Sucks!!!!!!!!!!!!!!!!

Just give me a break. I can't think about this. I am sick of my wheels turning, I'm sick of thinking. I'm just gonna try to chop some veggies for dinner and watch TV. I'm just going to forget it... for now. I wanna forget it forever. RE-WIND!

Have appt. with medical oncologist (chemo doctor) in London [on] Thursday, so she'll be able to say what showed up on CT scans the other day.

My appt. with the surgeon isn't till Nov 27th and he's on vacation so no point in pursuing that route.

OK, I'm done. I'm over it. I'm chopping veggies.

posted by Sarah @ 2:12 PM   6 comments

CHOPPING VEGGIES, THE CURE FOR CANCER?

See, I said it would all be better tomorrow and it was. No use in getting riled up unless there is absolute cause.

Friday I had my follow-up with the medical onc (chemo doctor) in London. I was expecting bad news that there was a tumour growing in my brachial plexus nerves because this is what they basically told me to expect. It would account for the loss of mobility in my wrist, fingers, elbow and severe nerve pain for which I now take: Methadone, Percocets, OxyContin, and Gabapentin... that's gotta give me some kind of street cred, no? I'm a hard-core junkie now!

Well, turns out, their guess was wrong! I am NED according to my recent scans! Yay, Sarah might get a break for a while! That lump I found last week is likely a seroma, but if it doesn't go away by my next appt Nov 27th then we'll do a needle biopsy and get it out if it is cancer. Just wait and watch. I'm soooo excited that I can actually start thinking about having a great Christmas... first of all that I will actually be ALIVE for it, and second of all that I likely won't even be sick for it! Sweet! This is the third Christmas I have been blessed with since cancer, and every one has had that cloud over it (will it be my last?) but at least I have great reason to believe that I will be here this year and I am so excited about looking forward to something!

I asked about my staging and they are considering me stage 4 rather than 3C at this point. Moving from stage 3 to stage 4 for a cancer patient is indescribable. We all DREAD the thought that that could one day be us. We hope, barter, bargain, pray, believe, that we can maybe just remain stage 3 forever.... Stage 4 is a whole other ball game. If you google stage 4 you don't find many happy stories, not with melanoma. But, it is NOT a death sentence!

I plan on living and not dwelling on what may or may not be. I am here NOW and I feel good NOW and cannot even begin to say how grateful I am for everything and everyone in my life. Not even 30, really just "starting out", but you know what? I've had it good. I have it good. I have such a true love in my life, my living angel who I have been blessed with for 9 years already! How many people get to say that? How many people have such a great core group of friends, who you know will be there for you no matter what, through sickness and in health? I've done a lot. And I plan to do a lot more. I just can't plan on time any more. Time is absolutely up in the air, so I must do things as the opportunities arise, as the money comes in, as I feel like it, without jeopardizing my husband's financial future at the same time somehow. Carpe Diem.

I decided this weekend that I want to volunteer. I can't have kids? So, I'll help kids. I'm going to look into after school home-work clubs, babysitting at women's shelters, and of course, because it's that time of year, helping with Christmas toy drives/food bank! That's the project for this week! I'm so excited at the prospect of having something to "do" for a few hours a week that will make me feel productive and hopefully fulfilled while helping children too.

I am so blessed to have a job that I can be on long-term disability and not have to worry too much about my income while I'm off. I get about 75% of my pay, so it's doable. For now, work is so on the backburner I don't even think of it. It was where I was. I am not there anymore and life has changed paths so I must forge through and clear the brush instead of getting stuck in the mud with nowhere to go. That was an old dream. My new dream is to just BE. And I have the LUXURY of being able to BE because of my insurance benefits. I am so lucky for this; so many people in similar circumstances don't have benefits for their drugs, work at fast-food places for minimum wage and have to think about their most basic needs on top of cancer. I am clothed, sheltered, sup-ported, financially OK, and can just BE and enjoy life.

posted by Sarah @ 10:38 AM   5 comments

A PICTURE IS WORTH A THOUSAND WORDS

This is gory so viewer beware.

I had my homecare nurse take some pics of my war wounds yesterday. The wounds from the Nov 2nd surgery got infected and re-opened once the steri-strips came off two weeks post-op. I believe the infection came about because of the steroids they put me on to prevent inflammation, combined with the fact that I have no lymph nodes left in the area to fight infection. But, the wounds from the other 2 surgeries, only weeks before healed up no problem. The difference is the steroids. The nurse must now visit me every day to "pack" the holes left on my body with gauze and clean out the area. It will be at least another 2 weeks of this until the holes heal up. It looks much worse than it is, I feel no pain. Possibly (OK, likely) because of all the pain meds I'm on for the nerve damage to my brachial plexus.

This [Pic 1] is my slashed (3 operations to remove tumours), and burned (radiation) axilla. It's got 1 long scar and some damaged skin. The pic is unfortunately kind of dark. My most recent scars [Pic 2] are on my shoulder (hole now), and side (chest wall). This pic [Pic 3] shows 2 that are totally healed and 2 that are still healing. The redness is just from the bandages irritating my skin.

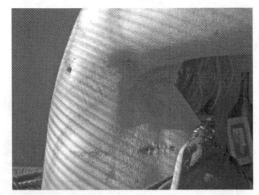

Pic 1

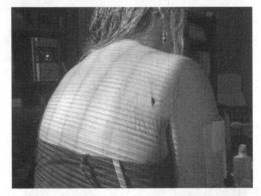

Pic 2

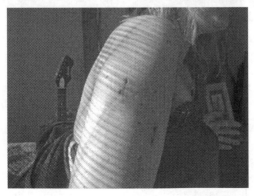

Pic 3

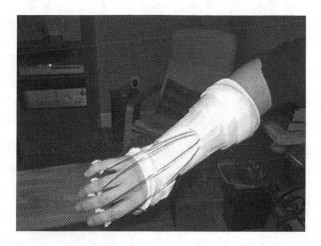

I still have complete loss of mobility of my right wrist and my fingers don' t work properly. They don't know if I will get mobility back, with nerve damage they can't predict apparently. I saw an OT (occupational therapist) and she made me this wicked contraption that helps to mobilize my wrist and the wires attached to my fingers help me move them! It looks CRAZY but it is sooo cool. I am typing right now with both hands which I haven't been able to do in a few weeks! I can write again and do just about anything when I wear this thing. It looks far more cumbersome than it is, I honestly barely notice I'm wearing it. It is far more uncomfortable not to wear it because then I notice the loss of function. The OT literally made the brace from scratch in front of my eyes over 3 visits and I am so grateful for it! I can brush my teeth again normally and put a clip in my hair! Still can't manipulate a hair elastic, but hey, I can use a knife, sign my name and do my zipper up again! Such little things, but it means so much to be able to do them again – who cares if I have to wear the bionic arm! I think it is fan-friggin-tastic!

I have been feeling really good the past couple of weeks. My pain is totally under control and I don't feel tired or loopy. The meds are doing their thing without changing my personality so I am quite pleased that we seem to have finally found the right mix at the right dose. Feeling so good means that I have TIME to do things, yet I'm not working. So, I did reach out and contact some agencies to volunteer and I am looking forward to it.

I met with the local hospice and I will be a volunteer driver for them. What that means is that they can call me to arrange to pick up a person who is terminally ill to bring them from home to the hospice for a program. The hospice offers free treatments like massage, Reiki and other programs to terminally ill people, but sometimes these people have no way to get to the hospice. So, they can call me and I can take them! They have to do a police check on me (oh, oh! what will they find?!) which will take a couple of weeks, then I will start getting calls. I'm really looking forward to meeting the clients. I will also be working a couple of shifts wrapping Christmas gifts on behalf of the hospice at the mall down the road. I LOVE gift wrapping. Weird, I know, but seriously, wrapping is my favourite part of Christmas! I love making pretty packages so I am looking forward to these wrapping shifts. The mall is in a community called Cherry Hill which is basically a geriatric neighbourhood. I mean, retirement community. I think the gift wrapping table at the mall will be well frequented by little old grannies with arthritis so I should be pleasantly busy making beautiful packages!

I also contacted a children's organization (which shall remain nameless because I don't want my blog to pop up when the organization is googled) and am working in a school one lunch hour per week helping with a sort of "good citizen" group for kids. I did it this week and it was a total gong-show. The woman running it was a wack-job and has no idea how to relate to kids, keep them interested, listen to them ... she was so out to lunch! I couldn't believe how the hour with 20 kids was squandered away because she was utterly disorganized, ill-prepared, and in another world.

The kids didn't seem to notice (they were between about 7-10 years old) and I think genuinely like her because she is "nice" but the group was chaotic and mostly they just talked amongst themselves while the woman rambled about home safety. I debated whether or not to return next week because I was so embarrassed to be a part of this group, but I'm going to give it another shot and see how much I can influence the woman and maybe help to run the program better.

Not to flatter myself but seriously, I could easily run the whole hour myself with very little preparation – it reminded me of the days when I was a camp counsellor and swim instructor. That was over 10 years ago now, but I was amazed how quickly I could get back into that mode and instruct kids. The thing is that this woman has apparently been running this group for a long time, and I'm just there to help. So, I don't want to step on any toes. She's just a volunteer though too. I'm going to try to wiggle my way in and make up for her deficiencies, because the kids deserve better, and the parents who have signed their kids up for this program deserve better. The manager of the organization called me and left a message saying I was apparently a "hit" with the kids and said if I wanted to speak with her I could call. I think she wants to know what I thought and also if I will stick around. I'm going to avoid talking with her until I've decided what to do. I feel weird just attending once and wanting to say that the program seemed to be an utter waste of time and the volunteer running it was clueless how to relate to kids, doesn't explain things well, didn't actually have a plan for the hour and wasted about half the time just thinking to herself out loud while the kids talked amongst themselves. I could have done better given 15 minutes prep-time if I was permitted to! But, it isn't my place. We'll see. I'll give it another shot; maybe it was just a bad day.

Blah blah blah. Going to meet some co-workers for lunch. They aren't going to recognize me with my steroid induced "moon face" and bionic arm! My face looks like a chipmunk from the steroids but I stopped them two days ago so hopefully the swelling will start to go down quickly! I can't stand my double chin.

In cancer related news, I have been avoiding "looking" for lumps and bumps so I have not found any new ones. My next appt. is Dec 1st at which time I will hopefully get the lump, that may or may not be a seroma, biopsied (it's growing actually instead of shrinking which is ominous but I'm in numb-mode so I don't worry about it). I'll look for other lumps the night before. No point in finding anything any sooner. Not that I would. I wouldn't dare find anything else. I'm getting a break. A long break from cancer.

posted by Sarah @ 12:08 PM   9 comments

I'M AN OLD PRO AT THIS

Well, I got a small break from surgeries, if not cancer alto-gether. My supposed seroma seems to be melanoma. The lump has grown from almond size to, wait, let me feel it....small plum size, in 3 weeks. It grew from nothing (my surgery Oct 3rd cleared out that area) to small plum size in 2 months. My mela-noma grows fast. Too fast for my liking, but I have no control over it. There is also a smaller lump, let's call it peanut size since we're on a food theme, right underneath it, hiding beneath my drain scar from one of my Oct surgeries. Derek and I went on a lump hunt (not quite as fun as an Easter egg hunt) last night and found nothing else, so I'm happy about that. The other thing to be happy for is that my surgery is this Tuesday! Man, the service just gets faster and faster at my cancer centre. I was in the right place at the right time, they had a hole to fill in the OR sched-ule so they stuck me in. I'll be hunky dory for the Christmas party we're hosting at home for friends on the 22nd as well as Christmas and New Year's unless something crazy happens... so all is well.

Got my path report back from the Nov 2nd surgery. There were 6 lumps taken out. One was not melanoma but plain old fatty tissue. To my surprise, the small lump in my breast was melanoma. Not the most common place for mm (malignant mela-noma) to spread, but it does happen. Now I can say I have had the exact same procedures as most early stage breast cancer pa-tients: lumpectomy, lymph node dissection, radiation with com-monly resulting lymphedema, just the procedures aren't in the same order! So, including the 2 masses that will be removed on Tuesday, that is 14 tumours removed in 2 months. Shitacular! OK, Sarah, focus on the positive. If you were in a third world country you would be dead by now and none of them would have been removed. My body has kept this disease out of my organs for over 11 years. I know it can continue to do it for many, many more! I have too much to live for and I love this life too much to move on just yet. UNIVERSE, DO YOU GET THE MESSAGE?!!!!

In non-cancer news: I went back to the school and it was much better. The woman, let's call her Doris, seemed somewhat more together. I haven't decided if that's because she had a cold last week and it made her brain foggy (too many antihistamines?) or if it's because the kids were busy making Christmas cards for some elderly adults in the community so she didn't need to talk much or keep the kids' attention. I wasn't paying much attention either to what she was doing because I was occupied touring around checking on how everybody was coming along and helping out with spelling, so it could be that I just didn't notice if she was still out to lunch.

Anyway, it went well and I really enjoyed the time around all the kiddos, watching them be creative and work as a team. It's so funny to watch the personalities come out, the bossy kid, the whiner, the tattle-tale, the peace-maker, etc. I wondered on the way home why I didn't become an elementary school teacher. Then I remembered – I only got a 3 year degree instead of 4 year and I cornered myself by taking a major that I hated (English lit.) and a minor (psychology) that I liked but to turn it into a major and continue on with my 4th year, I would have had to take more science oriented psych classes and Sarah doesn't do science. I sucked at it all through elementary and high school. I also had a fear that I would have to sing. Yup, like, la la la, sing. Don't all elementary teachers break out into song for class "fun"? At the very least around Christmas they make their classes sing carols. That's what it was like when I went to school anyway and I used to think that I would be forced to sing with my class if I was a primary teacher. I'm not a great singer. That's why I became a tax auditor.

Well, it's Friday and I have a wild night of making some kind of yummy baked treat and watching What Not To Wear [on TV] planned so I better get to it! Happy weekend to whoever is reading.

posted by Sarah @ 7:40 PM   6 comments

CURIOUS, QUITE LIKE GEORGE

So, you all know about me. I am so curious to "meet" all you cyber lurkers reading this blog. I get about 40-60 hits a day on this site (nothing compared to the 1 – 2 million perezhilton.com [a celebrity gossip website] gets!). Some of you I know IRL [in real life] and some of you I know from other message boards, and some of you have been sweet and courageous enough to introduce yourselves, but who are the rest of you?

This is your chance to come out of hiding. If you want to remain anonymous, that's cool, but just tell me a wee bit about yourself, like where you're from, if you have a similar story, or if you collect pet rocks. Just click on "comment" at the end of this entry and press "anonymous" if you aren't registered with Blogger.com.

I know most of you are from the States, followed closely by my fellow Canadians, then I get hits from the Netherlands (shout out Janette!) and the UK, sometimes Africa and Asia, but that's all I know about you! Can't blame me for being curious. Indulge me. I dare ya!

I'll start by telling you the latest about me. I had surgery on Tuesday to remove that area that they told me was likely a seroma from past surgeries in the same location. WRONG! It was a tooma, small plum size like I said, with a small almond size one beside it. I thought I found something on my shoulder too the day before the surgery so I called the secretary to let the surgeon know, see if he wanted to bring an ultra sound into the OR. That didn't happen so on the OR bed I had to decide if I wanted him to cut into me not knowing if there was anything bad there or not.

The surgeon's comment was that, "You are usually right about these things", which isn't really true. I'm sometimes right, sometimes paranoid. So, I had him cut in, just cuz it doesn't really hurt afterwards, and my shoulder, arm, armpit are so butchered already, what's another scar? Turns out he didn't find anything. Good. I'd rather know NOW then wait and watch and worry, especially over Christmas.

So, I will still be ship shape for Christmas unless shit hits the fan, but lets be optimistic. It's unlikely shit will hit the fan between now and New Year's, but I also know the reality from seeing how fast things have changed for some of my online melanoma friends. I know I am not exempt from this. I hope, but I am no more special or deserving than these wonderful people. We are all the same, just trying to get by, just hoping we will be on the good side of the stats. And we hope for each other.

posted by Sarah @ 2:20 PM   41 comments

ACTUALLY, IT'S DECEMBER 21ST WHEN I POSTED THIS ENTRY!

Edited to add: This is such a rambling incoherent mess. Not a reflection of my mind or how I feel, I just can't express my thoughts well. I started this entry on the 14th and saved it as a draft but didn't finish until I made myself tonight (21st). Been soooo busy! Fun busy though.

The other day, as I told a story in my cancer support group, I was reminded that I have been meaning to tell this story in my blog for ages, lest I forget, but really, how could I ever forget this, even with my atrocious memory?

In early September 2004 I got out of the shower one morning and found a golf ball sized lump in my armpit. The weather was warm and I was shaving the area frequently (unlike in the winter when I become a Sasquatch). I didn't think much of it as I had no idea it could be such an ominous sign of serious disease, I attributed it to a "swollen gland" due to a terrible cold. When it didn't go away for a few days, they started me on antibiotics. When that didn't work, a long two weeks of back and forths between my GP and emerg started, trying to figure out what this thing was. No one ever mentioned the C word, I was blissfully unaware, I thought at worst it was a cyst. Anyway, that's not the story, just the background and if you've been reading my blog you already know that.

So one day while I was still in the dark as to what this lump was, I was sitting on the toilet, minding my own business (while doing my business!) when probably the most surreal, inexplicable thing happened. As clear as can possibly be, a voice said to me:

"Hopes and dreams are just an illusion; all we have is the present."

I'm sure it was a male voice, a voice that entranced me. It was in my head, or in my ear, but it wasn't from me, if that makes sense. I knew that someone was speaking to me, I knew that this was a message that I had to remember, but I didn't know what the hell it meant. When I finished my business I wrote the sentence in a notebook which I still have because I knew I wouldn't remember but somehow knew this was something so important, I had to remember.

Soon, it became so clear. And this message is what I have referred back to over and over through this journey with cancer. When I got the final verdict by phone, "The cells are highly suspicious for malignant melanoma. I'm sorry, sometimes bad things happen to good people", and processed what I had been told over the next few days, or maybe weeks, the message made sense to me.

Everything we hope for, every dream or goal, that vision in our heads of how we think and therefore expect our life will be (give or take a few setbacks) is an illusion. Suffering occurs when our dreams for the future are crushed, but these dreams were never real and never guaranteed anyway so mourning their loss and suffering over it is really, really...silly.

This is a Buddhist teaching I believe, but at the time, I don't know that I was familiar with any Buddhist material really. Maybe I had read something to that effect and it was bubbling up subconsciously but I don't think that exact phrasing is from any text. Correct me if I'm wrong. And even if this did bubble up from my unconscious mind, the timing was bizarre, and I didn't even "get it" at the time; so what was my unconscious point?

When you get cancer with a bad prognosis, or any disease or life altering tragedy strikes, the real suffering is in mourning the loss of what you believed your life would be. For me, that was the job and course I was taking, the house I wanted to buy, the kids I wanted to have, the travelling, the grey hair, the grandkids. Typical stuff. But I could see it all so clearly, and even though I knew there would be bumps in the road and life would challenge me and offer up unexpected paths, I just knew that everything would be OK. I've had some terrible things happen in my life and I knew that bad things did happen to good people. But because I so clearly understood that my job was to mother and I could visualize my life through the decades as if they already existed. I was pretty much convinced that I would live a long life. [That's] more or less how I thought it would be.

I was also just beginning to realize at the time that I was living for the future. I was somewhat stuck in the "Everything will be good when X happens", but then X would lead to Y and Y would lead to Z and so on. Not that I wasn't happy, but I was always looking towards the future (do! do! do!), when things would be better instead of truly embracing the present and living. And what I've discovered is that living isn't doing, living is being.

I've said many times since this cancer journey began that I've done more living in the past two years than I have in my entire life. This isn't because I've all of a sudden had a lifetime of experiences, but because I've experienced and interpreted life in a different way, allowing me to take more of it in. I know, it sounds so cliché. But it is so true. I'm not going to ramble about what life feels like or looks like now because I wouldn't know how to explain it. It is just richer now; I see and feel things all the time now that I only got glimpses of before. I hate getting all "spiritual", not because I'm not, but because "spirituality" has almost become a cheesy commodity in recent years and I don't want to be perceived as a total flake. My spirituality is deeply personal and I would feel almost violated if I shared that part of myself with strangers.

All I will say is that something spoke to me that day. I don't know who and I don't care who, but it was nice of them. I don't believe I was supposed to "learn a lesson", I believe I was being comforted and reminded that life is now so I better not waste it wallowing in the "if onlys" and "why me's". Sure, I'm human and I do go there now and again, I especially did in the beginning of this disease, but when I go there, I have that phrase to remember, to shake me out of the self-pity. Hopes and dreams are just an illusion. I don't want to DO, I want to BE. That is living in the present. Being OK with being instead of doing, doing, doing. All we have is the present.

Cancer update: A few days after my last surgery (Dec 5th) I

found a pea size lump in my right breast. In October, one of the lumps I had removed was from my breast so I knew the melanoma had already spread there but I wasn't planning on finding more so soon. I guess I wasn't as thorough on my lump check pre-surgery as I thought I was, I think I totally ignored the boobs! I see my onc on January 8th for a follow-up and knew there was no way he'd call the office and roll me into surgery so soon after my last one to take one sub-q out so I'm just waiting. If it comes out, my bet is late January to February. I don't think about it, except that in the past couple of days I feel a little pressure in the area because it is growing and now it's probably the size of a large grape. It grows so fast! It's amazing how when I found this lump, I didn't even react. My heart didn't flutter, my stomach didn't jump. It was more just like, OK, been there, done that, whatever. I can't be bothered to get worked up over these tumours all of a sudden. They aren't specifically life-threatening and while I would like a break forever, it ain't happening at the moment so I've got to march forward and march through. Life will go on despite these little fuckers in my tissue. I guess because the sky hasn't dropped, my experience with these tumours has been OK, despite their overall significance and ominous meaning.

Thank you to everyone who introduced themselves. It was so nice to "meet" you. Your energy and spirits have and will help me get through this. It is so touching to know that so many people care. Having this place to vent is truly therapeutic. I kind of feel like I am giving away some of my worries, letting others carry some of the weight by sharing myself with virtual others in this way. Kinda cool.

posted by Sarah @ 7:36 AM   4 comments

HAPPY HOLIDAYS 2006

January 1, 2006 we moved into our first house and here she is a year later! It's much larger than it looks because it is looong. It's a duplex (note the two mailboxes) and we rent the front unit to my dad while Derek and I live in the back apartment.

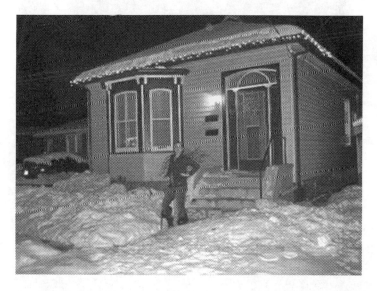

Here I am posing with the Christmas lights Derek put up (what a great job for his first time ever!) the day after our city got dumped on by the worst snowfall in 30 years. The city was shut down, even the transit system and every school. It's been such a wacky winter, we didn't have any snow accumulation before that day, it melted by the end of the week, and we haven't had any snow since! Yup, it was a green Christmas this year. But a great Christmas nonetheless!

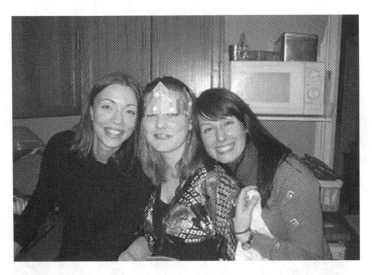

While in the middle of my steroid-induced "Euphoric Energizer Bunny" state that lasted from mid-November to early December, I had the bright idea of hosting a Christmas feast/party at our place for 17 people. I started to doubt my sanity as I slowly tapered off my steroids during December and felt my get-up-and-go slowly get up and go. I took my last dose the day before the party, and had enough umph still in me to pull it off virtually all by myself (thank God for Mom and her husband Dave who did all the chopping though!). It felt really good to be productive and self-reliant again – I had a lot of fun preparing and then eating and kickin' back with friends!

I know, you're wondering what on earth a vegan couple served to a mish-mash of omnivores, vegetarians, and one friend with celiac disease[18]. Well, I wanted to keep it really simple, so I made things that were easy peasy to prepare and served it buffet style:

---

18 Information about celiac disease is available at *www.celiac.com*

- Homemade hummus, baba ganoush and olive tapenade served with crackers (rice crackers for celiac) prepared the night before

- Rosemary and olive oil roasted potatoes

- Green beans roasted in raspberry balsamic vinegar and olive oil with dried cranberries and slivered almonds

- Mock "ham" (soy based) baked with pineapple slices – had many omnivores comment on how good the fake ham was!

- Mock "shrimp" ring (also made from soy) – again, even the real shrimp lovers were impressed!

- Cashew and poppy seed cabbage salad

- Portobello mushroom bake – I have to share this recipe because it is sooooo delicious, I think everyone should know about it.

- 3 pies. I made an apple pie and a chocolate mousse pie made with tofu that was literally to die for IMO [in my opinion], and I purchased a celiac-friendly walnut pie that was super scrumptious!

Portobello Mushroom Bake

1/2 c. almonds   1/4 c. olive oil

1/4 c. Braggs or soy sauce   1/4-1/2 c. water

2 tbsp balsamic vinegar   3 cloves garlic, roughly chopped

1 tsp dried rosemary   1 tsp dried oregano

1 medium onion, chopped

4 large Portobello mushrooms, cleaned and stems removed

Preheat oven to 350F. In a blender or food processor, blend the almonds until powdered. Add all other ingredients [except mushrooms] and blend until well combined. In a large baking dish, place mushrooms upside down and pour mixture evenly overtop. Bake for 20 – 25 mins. Makes 2 – 4 servings.

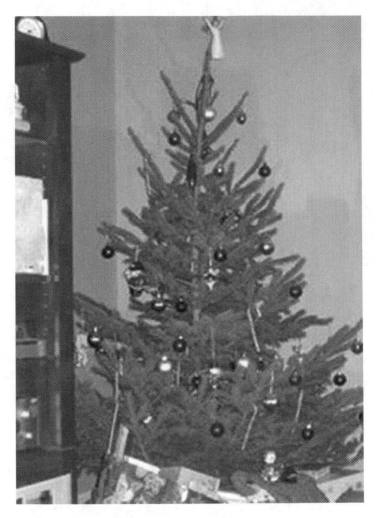

Our first Christmas tree. We picked it together. Derek chopped it down himself from a tree farm. Even though we've been living together for 7 years, we've never done the tree thing. I think it was the combination of it being our first house and the fact that I was soooo into the Christmas spirit this year that we did the tree, the lights, the party, and also for the first time exchanged stockings.

While it is my 3rd Christmas with cancer, it is the first one in that time that I've felt really well, even though technically, I'm much sicker. Last year sucked because I got the blow a couple of days before [Christmas] that I had my 1st recurrence (well, technically my second) and I was still getting my energy back after stopping interferon 2 weeks prior. I was on my way to Kingston with my brother by bus [to spend Christmas with my mom] and scheduled in an appt. with my onc during our layover in Toronto when I got the news. I gave my bro the gifts and hopped on a bus back to London because I needed the comfort of Derek's arms. He can make everything OK just with his embrace. The year before, I had just completed my high-dose [interferon] regimen and felt too crappy to travel to Kingston.

This year, my mom came to London for Christmas! Now that we have a house with a dining room we can do Christmas! And, we did do it, quite nicely I might add. Derek cooked the entire meal (minus the turkey for the meat-eaters) thank God because by the 25th I was feeling really crappy from the steroid withdrawal. I was tired, nauseated, bloated, and lethargic. He did a fantabulous job with dinner; I just wish I was able to enjoy it more. The rest of the fam (just mom, Dave, and my brother) sure enjoyed the feast though. Derek and I had a yummy Tofurky [available at health food stores, and larger grocery stores], in case anyone is wondering what we eat instead of birds on holidays.

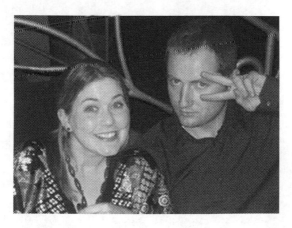

This is us on New Year's Eve in Toronto. You caught me, I'm wearing the same top that I wore at our party. All I can say is, I like it! It has flowy arms that hide my lymphedema quite nicely without being a big frumpy sweater.

I'm really not liking how fat my face is, I think it's because of the steroids. Well, I'm off them now so it should go down soon I hope. I don't recognize myself when I catch glimpses of myself in windows or store mirrors. At home, I don't notice as much. I've gained almost 10 lbs. since November and am at my highest ever weight because of it. I think it is because the steroids turned me into a ravenous pig for a few weeks while I was at the peak dose. The roundness of my face could be pure fat, but I am hoping it's the typical "moon face" that people get as a side effect of Decadron which goes away sometime after you stop.

Sure, it's all so trivial and so petty compared to what others go through. And I tell myself that. But the automatic thoughts are hard to push away. It's hard to look in the mirror and barely recognize yourself. It's hard to see the effects of cancer treatment so blatantly displayed in front of you. It's something I haven't had to deal with yet in my journey. All my scars can be hidden by clothes. But now, I have a big fat face for all to see and my right arm has ballooned even more since I've had those wounds that got infected and STILL won't heal.

In fact, I've had a homecare nurse come everyday to clean, pack and dress the wounds for a month and a half and while they were progressing slowly, it appears I have another infection and one wound that was 90% healed and didn't need special attention is now infected too bringing the count to 4. I find out tomorrow if I'm supposed to start IV antibiotics.

Anyway, I know I shouldn't care about how I look, but I do. I want to be attractive to my husband. I don't want to be a chubby, round faced, double chinned, fat-disfigured-armed, tumour ridden wife. He says I'm beautiful anyway, and I do believe him, but how the hell am I supposed to feel pretty and sexy inside when I'm not myself anymore? When my breast has a tumour again. When my wrist hangs limp and I can no longer straighten my elbow. When I can't do my hair nicely, can't even put it in a pony tail because I can no longer manipulate an elastic, hold a blow dryer or flat-iron. I have to wear baggy shirts so my arm isn't as noticeable. No more cute tops for me. I miss having showers and taking real baths. I can't get my wounds wet so I have quick uncomfortable and shallow baths and Derek washes my hair while I lean over the tub. This has been going on for months as I have surgery after surgery and now those damn wounds that won't heal. And more surgery likely to come. It would be so nice to lay back and relax in our deep clawfoot tub again.

I beat myself up even more for caring about these things. There are far worse problems in the world and people suffer much much more. But psychologically, I get it. With every new "loss", I go through a period of mourning until I am able to accept the new normal. I had more or less accepted the state of my arm until it recently got much worse and bigger. It will take a bit to adapt to the new larger state and the fact that I will never be able to whip my hair up into a pony-tail again. My weight gain makes me think mostly about how I can't just jump on the elliptical we bought in September or go for a run anymore. Maybe one day I'll work out again, but it has been really frustrating being forced to be so lazy the last few months with all the pain and then surgery after surgery. We should have bought a good recumbent bike instead of the elliptical because I think that would be fine on my arm and neck. We couldn't have known though.

God, I'm tempted to erase this because I feel like such a whiner. But I know it's natural to have these ups and downs. And I know it's OK, even if it isn't stoic or graceful, to mourn every loss that comes along. Just like I had to mourn the loss of many of my dreams, like having children. To be resistant to change is natural, especially changes that were forced upon me and which make life just that little bit more difficult when life seemed difficult enough. Having to give up even more control of my body is difficult to accept but I'll get there, it's a process and this whining is part of it.

Every Christmas, New Year's and birthday that passes since I've had cancer seems like a miracle because I know it could easily be my last, so much more so than the average person. I'm so thankful that I've now had 3 Christmas and soon 3 birthdays (pretty darn confident and hopeful I'll make it to Feb 7th, my 30th birthday!) since being diagnosed when it's always in my mind that it could be my last. This year more than ever, since I've progressed to stage 4, I am even more aware of the possibility that could have been my last Christmas. I think that that is really what was behind me "getting into the spirit" and pushing for a fun New Year's out instead of the usual house party or just staying at home. I want to have great times with family and friends and make sure I do things I want to do now instead of bowing out due to pure laziness and the knowledge that there is "always next year". I can't take that risk because I may not get the chance. In 2004, I was so unsure if I'd be around in 2005. I've made it to 2007, so much longer than many with this same disease. I'm so grateful for this time yet so scared my time is running out. I feel like a ticking time-bomb. I hate this fucking disease! One day at a time, I'm just trying to buy time until there is a cure.

posted by Sarah @ 4:36 PM   7 comments

THERE ARE SO MANY WORDS FOR VOMIT... WHICH ONE SHALL I USE?

I'm so tired. Sleeping is all I want to do. Felt the same last week up until the weekend when I somehow perked up for 4 days, drove 2 hours to Toronto, partied (lightly) for New Years. The day after we got back home, the fatigue set in again. Is it depression? Is my fibromyalgia back? It's been years since I've had a fibromyalgia episode.

I attributed the fatigue last week to steroid withdrawal but after my 4 days of chipperness I thought I was over it. Makes no sense. I'm scared something is really wrong. Do I have tumours near my heart, in my liver, somewhere else that would account for the fatigue? I don't know much about physiology.

I've been crying a lot. I guess that optimism, strength, cheerfulness, inspiration I had been feeling for a couple of months was steroid induced. It wasn't me, it was the drug... damn, that's a disappointment. I really hope the steroids weren't just masking this mood, but that this mood is just a withdrawal symptom. I could sleep 24 hours a day. But I have to get up for certain things, and to appear OK. Today I went to a movie with my dad. I nearly fell asleep. Napped from 11:30 am – 12:30 pm (had to get up for movie) and 4 pm – 9 pm then Derek woke me up. I made myself get up to eat something. I have no appetite, the thought of most things makes me queasy, but it is so important to stay nourished. I had PB&J [peanut butter & jam] on an English muffin, grapes and applesauce. Then I perked up enough to watch The Black Dahlia on DVD. I liked it, but found it really difficult to follow. Now it's 12:30 am and I'm about to pass out.

Had a CT scan today. See my surgeon on Monday and I hope he has some preliminary results at least. Of course, I'm scared shitless what they'll find. I know of 4 probable tumours: breast, shoulder, side, armpit... scared he won't or can't take them all out. Especially the one in the axilla. That area has been pushed to its limit. Unless they bring in a plastic surgeon, there is no tissue or skin left to stretch and sew back. And I don't want to be cut anymore. My breast will be mangled, my arm will get even bigger if they do the axilla. What if I get even more nerve damage? My arm is destroyed. I'm too embarrassed even to post a pic of what it has turned into: a big fat, limp and lifeless, deformed mess. But I suppose I should to document what I have been through. If I don't make it, at least this blog will still exist.

I don't know when to stop the cherry picking. But they do hurt once they reach a certain size and they grow at such an exponential rate they really can't be left in. But at what point do I try IL-2? Before I had said I wanted to cherry pick until it spreads to an organ and then I'd go to IL-2. But if I was one of the lucky 5% that gets a long remission or even one of the 20% who gets a short remission, I'd get a break, without getting more disfigured by surgery. But the treatment would make me unimaginably sick. I can't fathom going through it for an 80% chance I'll get no response. My brain hurts thinking about it. I'm so sick of being "sick". Yup, I'm throwing a fucking pity party and no one is invited because I'm too tired to socialize.

I want to do a combination therapy recommended by a naturopath either involving high dose vitamin C or mistletoe (or both) and a bunch of other supplements, but we just can't afford it. Mistletoe is the #1 alternative adjuvant treatment in Europe (google it, it's true) and while vitamin C by IV is controversial, even some doctors in the States prescribe it as a last resort. There are many many documented cases of complete remission in different diseases, not just cancer. But these are anecdotal cases and studies have not shown it to have significant survival benefit.

It costs $140/week or $50/week if I can find someone who

is willing to administer it to me intravenously outside the naturopath's office. I don't have any nurses in my family though and can't find anyone else. It sucks, because as if we can afford $140/week on top of the $200 – 300 [per month] we already spend on supplements. I know, I know, it sounds crazy, but because I've been alive for over 2.5 years since it recurred in my lymph nodes, and so far has only recurred in soft tissue and nodes, it's impossible to say whether or not the supplements have had a role in this. I can't just stop them, in case they have!

Well, this has been pleasant. Needed to vent more I guess. I feel like I just puked up all my worries (OK, a fraction of my worries) all over you. What a mess. I feel like I may have more to come though, so beware!

Goodnighty night.

posted by Sarah @ 12:06 AM   10 comments

JANUARY 16, 2007

I CHOPPED IT!

My hair hasn't been this short since 1993.

Finally had to take the plunge and do what makes sense since I can't really "do" my hair anymore, which really for me means sticking it in a pony tail.

I'm pleasantly surprised with the results and am relieved I can really just "wash and go" now.

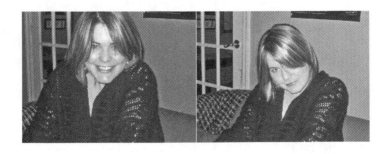

A serious blog update is in order but I just haven't felt like it. I have much of my energy back, but am still taking it easy cuz if I don't I get really tired. My appetite is much better but not nearly back to normal. I've only had one "real" dinner in 2.5 weeks, the other times it's cereal and banana or grapes and an English muffin, that sorta thing.

I'm off to my abdomen ultrasound. They sent me home yesterday because I told them I had a protein shake before coming. Oops, forgot my tummy was supposed to be empty. That was a

7:30 am appt. and my make-up today is at 9:30. Too bad I had to have a bowl of grapes to tide me over... My blood sugar gets really low and I get the shakes and get really weak (probably accounts for a good part of my fatigue the past couple of weeks since I haven't been eating consistently) and since I have to drive myself to the appt., then walk thru the hospital I just thought SCREW IT, I have to eat something! So I just won't tell the receptionist. I'm sure the ultrasound tech will see the mashed up grapes in my belly or wherever they have travelled to by 9:30 am but they'll just have to get whatever imaging they can considering. It was ordered by my surgeon because of my fatigue. Since I'm getting better, I'm pretty sure it was the 'roid withdrawal and the wound infection throwing my body off. Whatever.

Man, I have sooooo much to say but it makes me tired just thinking about it. I have to try and write it out this week before it never gets documented.

Shit, I'm gonna be late, I'll edit this later, there must be even more typos than usual!

posted by Sarah @ 8:46 AM   22 comments

BUFFALO REVISITED

Finally, I'm writing. Can't say that I really want to, but I have to before life slips by undocumented as I can't trust my terrible memory to store the details. I have a terrible memory and those who know me would probably say that's an understatement. I constantly forget details of friends' lives making me look like a bad listener or that I didn't care. It's not that at all, God, I can't even remember what happened to myself! It's a total information coding problem, I'm clearly brain-damaged so people just have to learn to love me for it and I have to learn to love myself despite this brain blip!

Don't ever ask me to review a movie for you. I can't. I can remember whether I like it or not but I can only remember the story line for a couple of days. Same with books. But I enjoy them nonetheless as momentary entertainment. My mom is the exact same way so whatever this problem is, it's hereditary and it gets worse with age. I started noticing my memory was going down hill at around 20 and in the last 10 years it's gotten to the point that people comment on it. Oops, how's that for a free-flowing rambling tangent? I really just seem to write what I'm thinking instead of thinking about what I'm writing. I guess that's the easy thing to do and I like easy. Oops there I go again...

It hurts physically to sit at the computer. It hurts more to type. I have to get my meds readjusted.

Man, this month has been physically and emotionally exhausting. I'm past the days of sleeping 18 – 20 hours a day and only eating grapes and walnuts. There was a couple of weeks there that if I wasn't in bed, I was on the couch and I was too tired to fix myself drinks or meals, not that I felt like eating anything. Think of the one food that repulses you so much you can't even imagine taking a bite of it. That's how I've been with ALL foods, and I loooove food! The only things I could stand to eat were grapes, walnuts, English muffins with margarine and honey, popsicles, mandarin oranges, yogurt, and sometimes Cheerios with banana and soy milk. It was a gradual progression to even get to that point though. In the beginning, it was just a few grapes and a couple of walnuts. Literally, that's all I could bear to eat in a day.

I'm proud to say that I've come a long way since even last week and today I had my Cheerios and banana for brekkie, an Amy's bean burrito for lunch, and some left over stir-fry on rice for dinner. I'm not enjoying my food, but at least I can tolerate it. I'm sleeping 11 hours/night but not taking naps so that's good. I'm tired but can go out if I have to for a bit.

No one can give me a reason why I've been feeling so shitty. The liver ultrasound was negative, I'm not pregnant, blood work doesn't show anything besides the fact that I'm mildly anaemic but so mildly it wouldn't account for such severe fatigue. Some say it could be from being off the steroids but others think that a month after the fact is far too late for me to still be having withdrawal symptoms. Other theories are depression and stress. I tend to think it is 100% steroid-related as it started right after I stopped the steroids (Nov/Dec were wonderful months filled with steroid induced über energy and euphoria). My fatigue is slowly getting better and happened before I got the stressful news that I am finally about to write about.

At the beginning of January I had a CT scan. The scan showed that my organs are clear (yay!) but that the disease has spread a lot in all the areas that have previously been affected and has also taken up shop in my brachial plexus. Yup, the same area that Toronto said had disease back in September but then London said it didn't, so I didn't do IL-2. Another scan in November confirmed that there was still no disease in the BP [brachial plexus] even though the loss of mobility in my arm and hand (radial nerve damage) suggested there might be. So, now it's official, it is there. It can't be removed, and there is a big tumour in my axilla that can't be removed. I also have TONS of other little areas of disease in that whole region. I can see and/or feel some of the tumours and others are there, just too small yet to see or feel.

My right breast has 4 tumours that I can feel and they are getting so big that they are starting to blend together so it almost feels like 3/4 of my breast is a rock. I've got others on the back of my shoulder and upper arm that are walnut sized and then at least 10 other pea size ones I can feel that by this time next month will be walnut sized. They are popping up like crazy and will continue to do so unless something stops it. Surgery can't stop this.

So, it's off to Buffalo for IL-2 (paid for by the Ontario gov't). I've explained in a previous post why I have to go to Buffalo so I won't get into that. It'll be sometime next month before that treatment starts, I'm guessing towards the end of the month but it's hard to say.

I wish I had the energy to write about … my medical onc in London, but it would take me forever to recount my last two meetings with her. I really want to like her because I'm caught between a rock and hard place in that she is the only onc in the city that deals with mel patients and I don't want to be travelling back and forth between home and some other city for my follow-up care.

I won't have to see her very much as I'll be treated in Buffalo but I presume I'll be seeing her for routine follow-up between treatments. I don't doubt that she can do that, it's just that … I know that everything she says has to be taken with a grain of salt and I'll have to verify her "information" on my own. Man, I wish I could write out the things she has said to me… things so off-base, delusional and/or rude that she has had me in tears and I mean big ugly sobbing tears because she was just so wrong in certain things and wouldn't hear otherwise. Such a power-tripper. It's her tone of voice, it's the way she words things. It's the stare. It's the whatever-I'm-saying-is-important-but-whatever-you-say-I'll-dismiss attitude. Fuck her.

My second meeting with her this month was basically a mediation session with the social worker to get me the information I didn't get in our last meeting while she was pursuing her own agenda and yapping. The social worker and I have decided that she (the social worker) will be attending all my future appointments with the medical onc so I can have a witness. The main problem is that the doctor will tell me something then later tell me she didn't say that, or tell me I told her something that I didn't. I feel like I'm in the twilight zone. Luckily Derek and my mom were in the first meeting so I had witnesses there to assure me it wasn't me that was crazy and they agree that she is a major piece of work who specializes in de-humanizing people. Today, the onc was on her best behaviour as her colleague was present but she still flip-flopped on what she said and managed to avoid answering basic questions such as "what are the different options for me at this point, and what is your recommendation?" until the question was re-phrased 3 times. Gah! Anyway, in the future, I have my back-up so it'll be alright. I don't have to like her. It would be soooo nice and I deserve to have better care but travelling [to Toronto] for it doesn't make sense when the options will be the same. If I need to go onto another treatment in the future then I will seek a second opinion for sure but if the treatment is offered in London then I'll have to deal with her.

Please, I don't need anyone from the U.S. telling me to go to M.D. Anderson or anywhere else. There is no way on earth I could afford to. Imagine if you had to pay 100% out of pocket for every visit, every test, every treatment and the air travel. Give me a break. The only thing the U.S. can offer that we don't have is a gazillion clinical trials (and lets face it, getting a good response out of clinical trial is like winning the lottery), routine PET scans (controversial anyway) and GAMMA knife for brain mets (in general only buys patients a few weeks/months anyway...yes, there are always exceptions!). So, for that it ain't worth going into debt $100,000 when the end result is almost always the same at this stage. I don't mean to be a pessimist and I believe there is always hope, but sometimes you have to take the reality of the statistics into consideration and consider the financial devastation you could be leaving a loved one with.

Wow, this has been a depressing entry. I'm gonna change it up a bit next time and do the entry that I really wanted to do, not the one I had to do just for updating sake. Since it's the new year and I think I have all my photos from last year on the computer, I want to upload pics from my favourite adventures of 2006.

posted by Sarah @ 6:15 PM   8 comments

CHECKING IN

I'm OK, just hurts my arm, neck, hand too much to type. Working on different pain med combos.

IL-2 in 2 – 3 weeks. Hopefully I'll be able to type more by next week.

posted by Sarah @ 1:42 PM   10 comments

IT'S NOT JUST A GRANDPA DISEASE

I didn't know this brave young woman from B.C. but her mother has posted on another site that, in her daughter's honour, she'd like to get her message out. Please take a moment to click the link below[19] and listen to Ceri's message, because even in death her voice is still strong and able to continue educating about skin cancer and the possible dangers of the sun.

R.I.P. Ceri Elizabeth Smith 1986 – 2007

posted by Sarah @ 9:47 PM   3 comments

---

19 *http://www.youtube.com/watch?v=miZHXxng9UE*

IT'S VALENTINE'S DAY

We don't do anything extravagant for v-day, but we do acknowledge it most years. Valentine's Day happens many times during the year at our house, any time one of us does something special for the other is romantic enough for this gal. I'm not the diamond necklace and roses kinda gal.

I had literally forgotten about v-day until last night. Or more accurately, I'd remember and panic, then forget again. In bed last night, Derek mentioned it was v-day tomorrow and I was like, holy shit, I didn't do anything for you, I forgot with everything that's been going on... I never seem to know what day it is. He said, No worries, I didn't get anything for you either. So, this morning D-man left for work at 8:50 am and I rolled out of bed at 10:30 am to find a cute basket filled with vegan/organic chocolates of different varieties, my favourite tea and another tea that looks yummalicious and some natural soaps. Aw, what a sneaky little sweetheart.

My plan is to make some vegan cupcakes with red or pink hearts on top. I've sent my dad out to get the icing and I'm nervous what he'll come home with. We are also out of sugar so I'm waiting for him to get back home this afternoon so I can borrow sugar. No, he doesn't exactly live with us, I think I've mentioned before that we own a duplex (a 100 year old house converted into two roughly 900 sq ft 2 bedroom apartments) and he rents one apartment from us. We live in the bigger one. So anyway, I hope I can finish these cuppy-cakes before Derek gets home. It's going to be quite the feat considering how much pain I've been in, which makes the cupcakes extra special because he'll know how painful it was to make them. But he deserves it and when there's a will, there's a way. I don't necessarily believe that cliché but in this particular circumstance, it works!

So, I'm back blogging. With one hand mind you. That equals slow blogging. Derek got a great deal on a used laptop for my birthday on Feb 7th and I just called today to get the wireless connection and am so excited at the prospect of lying on the couch or in bed catching up on emails and stuff. Sitting at the desktop is painful for me in my back and neck, and if I try using my right hand, even with my bionic arm, I get terrible pain in my arm cuz I have to reach up too far for the keyboard.

Ya, so my 30th birthday was on the 7th. It was definitely different than I had pictured it growing up. Like most people, I think, I thought of it as this huge milestone in life, worth celebrating with a huge party. And then behind closed doors I thought I'd wrestle with all the feelings that I thought go along with this milestone. You know, like feeling old and needing to assess where my life was at and if I had achieved everything I had wanted to achieve in my dream or illusion of what my life was supposed to be like by age 30. I actually did pretty well on the checklist. That sort of unwritten checklist I think lots of people share, unless I'm just crazy. The checklist that meant you were truly a self-sufficient adult. I wanted to get there, some people avoid it like the plague and want to remain free of responsibility, living sort of free of commitment, never really aging mentally. But I had that checklist and it involved working towards, and hopefully achieving, the following things by the time I was 30:

- Finish degree and commit to life-long learning – I don't want to become stagnant.

- Find a job that I didn't hate and that would allow me to be self-sufficient, with benefits.

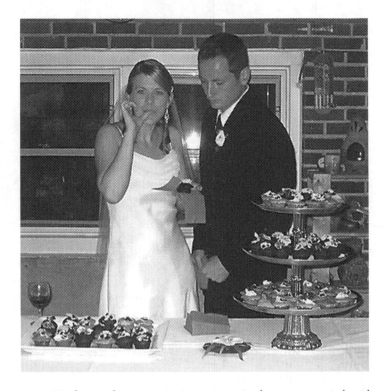

- Find a quality partner. I never wanted to get married and I don't really believe that humans need to commit to each other for life. This is sort of like the Buddhist teaching of impermanence: Everything changes, and if we can't accept that things change or go away then that leads to suffering. How can we possibly know that 20 years from now we'll want to be with the same person? People develop and expand at different speeds. Why commit to someone for life when this could lead to personal misery? Most people just get divorced these days or literally suffer through a platonic relationship for years because of this commitment in front of God. Of course there are many exceptions and this is merely my opinion. But as we both saw it, we were on a journey together, a ride that we got on and couldn't know when the ride would end, if ever. Why not just go with the flow? Of course, all the time hoping that our partnership would last our lifetimes. Neither of us have qualms about having children out of wedlock. And we had already made it 7 years when I realized we needed to get married. Derek thought I was joking. We got married because no one took us seriously when we said, "This is my boy/girlfriend." They didn't know if we had only been together for 3 weeks so we had no right to speak on each other's behalf. Derek had no right to advocate for me in medical situations. Now he can. Doctors talk to him if I'm drowsy, etc., and take him seriously and allow him to speak on my behalf and make decisions. It came down to we were ambivalent about marriage, so why not just do a very secular wedding and throw a backyard party. It was also a sneaky way to get ALL our friends across the country to be in the same place at the same time.

- Buy a house.
- Have a baby.

So, I did everything except have the baby, but it doesn't really matter because I have cancer. Yes, I'm blessed to have such comfort and security having long-term income protection and heath benefits. I'm so blessed to have the best husband in the world who friggin' does everything for me if I'm feeling shitty or in pain. He makes sure I'm comfy, cleans the house, literally comes home from work, asks me about my day, starts dinner, and fixes up the house before he gets to relax. It's not fair. But he says he doesn't mind, refuses my thanks and still showers me with kisses and caresses. I said the other day how sorry I was that we haven't made love in so long due to surgeries and pain and my hang-ups about being ugly with visible tumours and he said something like, "I don't care about that at all. We make love everyday in different ways. Sex is such a small part of what makes our relationship, so please don't worry about that." Sorry if that was TMI [too much information] but I wanted to document that for myself. See what a sweetie-pie he is? I'm sooo lucky! That doesn't mean we don't have spats once in a while, but it seems that when I'm sick or in pain he kicks it up a notch and we don't argue. Probably too, cuz

I don't have the energy to nag. I'm pretty darn lucky to have him. How could I possibly go through this without him? It would be truly horrific.

Woops, I went on a tangent. I'm trying to make a point and that is, I don't feel old, I feel too young to have cancer. Too young to have to face such torture and pain. So many people hit 30 and freak about the number's significance to them. I thought I was going to be like that, but since I was dx'd at 27 I have just begged the universe to let me live that long. It seemed so far into the future considering the terrible statistics that went along with my dx. Was I, could I, possibly make it to that marker? And I did! And instead of wanting to party about it (believe me, I was in no state to party anyway) I just kinda wanted to sit with it, be grateful for it. Derek made me a vegan chocolate cake and I got visits from friends and family with prezzies[20] and flowers. It was perfect and I can't see it being any other way…low key is my new status. And ya know what? If I can do 3 years then I can do 3 more and keep running with it! I'm back in cancer ass-kicking mode and this IL-2 will work for me!

In other cancer news:

Still waiting for my IL-2 date. I was so hoping it would be this Monday (19th) because I have had all the tests and scans done.

I'm worried that my scans weren't good and they are thinking about palliative alternatives. I hope hope hope that in the month since my last scan things haven't drastically changed. Yes, I've called the doctor, talked to her nurse who had no idea London was taking care of things cuz the last thing she heard was that Toronto was doing all the paper work. She asked me if I had the results of the scans to which I said no and she said she'd talk to Dr. G and call me back. That was yesterday afternoon. I'm going to harass her again as soon as I finish this entry. Edit to add: I got word today that I will get a letter in the mail tomorrow saying I have an appt. within 7 days for Buffalo. I think the letter will have the exact date. Woohoo!

We went to Ottawa this weekend (Fri – Mon) and stayed in a cute hotel called the Bostonian[21] which had only suites with

---

20 Sarah-ism meaning "presents"
21 Bostonian Executive Suites, 341 Maclaren St., Ottawa – 866-320-4567

full kitchen – I'm talkin' dishwasher too! And only $110/night, a kilmometre walk to the parliament buildings and many of the attractions Ottawa has to offer. We saved a lot of moola cooking our own food, and Granny, who lives in Ottawa paid for the suite as well as my dad. Very nice of them to allow us this mini vacation. We were concerned about my pain level but decided it would be "funner" to be in pain at a hotel than at home. Saturday, I exceeded my expectations and was out and about doing the tourist thing a good part of the day. I was in pain the whole time but with breaks I was able to go on. Sunday though was a whole other story. I couldn't get comfortable during the night cuz now it is getting increasingly hard to even sleep on my left side cuz of pain. My left side was the only position I've been able to semi-sleep in for a month. By the morning, I knew I was out of commission for the day, possibly because I over did it the previous day. Derek went exploring by himself for a few hours while I slept. At bed-time, I was in so much pain I was rolling around crying and being a total bitch because Derek wanted to help so bad but there was nothing he could do... I just wanted to try to find a position on my own. After about an hour of this I said, I'm going to emergency, I can't take this. So we took a cab to the hospital, I was triaged in like 30 seconds. It's amazing how fast you get in when you say "stage 4 cancer pain". I'm thinking some dude out there with a broken leg waiting for 4 hours to see a doctor could be in just as much pain as me and I get in so fast? It's not fair, but as if I would speak up and risk losing my spot! Anyway, we decided that I would stay overnight so I could get IV morphine every 1/2 to 1 hour (which just took the edge off enough to get a bit of shut-eye for an hour or two at a time). Derek went back to the hotel to get a little sleep. This was at 3 am mind you. It took so long because there was a trauma they had to take care of first. You should have seen Derek's eyes, they were so bloodshot cuz he was so tired, sitting in a regular office chair for 4 hours but all he cared about was me. God, I HATE doing this to him. But I'd be screwed without him. No one knows how to take care of me but him.

Obviously pain meds aren't working. Pain onc has been fiddling with my meds ever since they stopped working about 3 weeks ago. Nothing is working. Every 3 or 4 days we change something, double something. Nope, not good. Can't sleep, can't drive, can't cook, can barely get dressed, can't clean. How's that for quality of life? If what I'm on now doesn't work by tomorrow morning, then I am likely going to some kind of drip. A tube will be inserted into me, attached to a little baggy that is programmed to regulate dosage. Not sure what drug. I don't like the idea of it just like I didn't like visible tumours on my body. I want to avoid looking like I have cancer so I don't have to identify with it. In my mind, I am a healthy person, healthier than most people, the doctors even refer to me as a "healthy girl" – hey, now that I'm 30 should I insist on being called a healthy woman? – except this physiological error happened, something that is not a part of who I am. I feel invaded and I feel it wasn't meant to happen. Ah, well, I must do whatever will make me comfortable until we annihilate this nasty, unwanted, disease from my body! I'll get over the bag within a few days I'm sure.

Tumours are taking over. No longer just on my right side, the cancer has made a home in many different places and I feel a new tumour almost every day. My left neck, my stomach, my upper groin area, my back, more on the right side. That was heavy news to swallow when I felt the first one in a place other than my right armpit, shoulder, arm or breast. Whatever though, I'm still fighting this beast down to the ground. I will be on the good side of the stats. Why the hell not? Now I just wish my medical "team" treated me like that was possible too.

I think that's it. The fact that I even wrote this is a sign of progress. But, it really ain't fun typing with one hand. My totally sincere apologies to any one I owe email responses to. I literally have only been logging on to the old 'puter once or twice a week and not for long because of pain so I try to respond to emails by earliest date. I think it'll be much better when the wireless laptop is hooked up sometime next week.

Gotta go finish those cupcakes – eek, the bottoms got slightly burned, but it's the thought that counts! I'm no Martha. Nor do I want to be.

posted by Sarah @ 1:19 PM   17 comments

JUST CALL ME THE ONE-HANDED WONDER

Tisk, tisk. With my memory I should be blogging more regularly. But, ya do what you can do, yo.

Is it actually March first? I don't like how time flies. Especially when I'm somewhat sidelined and unable to do as much as I'd like to do with my time. I hate saying it, but the last 2 months haven't consisted of much more than dragging myself out of bed between 10 am – 1 pm, then plopping myself on the couch for the rest of the day to watch TV, read, make phone calls (usually related to medical or supportive care, meaning social work or group, that kinda thing). Up until the last 2 or 3 weeks, I was able to drive so I could take myself to this or that appointment but I've lost that independence now. For real excitement, I'd have over a couple of visitors a week (too much socializing drains me), watch DVDs on weekend nights with friends. All because of PAIN!

I don't know where exactly I got the idea that most cancer pain was manageable. Like so many other impressions I had about cancer until I was thrown into this life, I just recently realized that my impression, while not untrue, was a bit simplistic, or a bit black and white. My cancer pain can be managed, but not with a decent quality of life. I still feel like I can and should have a relatively normal lifestyle... going out for dinners, shopping for fun OR necessity (I wish I could go grocery shopping!), having some drinky poos with friends. I feel mentally and physically ready for this, minus the pain.

Here's the stab at the heart: In order for my pain to be completely under control, I'd be a zombie!

I kept returning to the cancer centre saying, "This isn't working". So they'd up the doses as far as they could without nasty side effects occurring. It wasn't until a couple of weeks ago that I got the nerve to ask what their goal was for me pain-wise. In my head, I totally thought we were working to get me to the point I described above. But just in case, I didn't ask. Their answer broke my heart (how many times can a heart get broken?). They said they wanted to get me into a "comfortable resting state", which I took to mean comfy on the couch. And the truth was, I was pretty much comfortable on the couch in certain strategic positions. But I wasn't ready for that. That's not my life, not now. Believe it or not, I still think of myself as a healthy person! Call me sick, and I think, "But I don't have a cold."

So, along came the CADD [Continuous Ambulatory Drug Delivery] pump this week which is a rectangular box, about 9x2 inches and weighs like 2 lbs. Part of the contraption holds my medication (Dilaudid) which flows through a tiny plastic tube, through a small needle, and into my sub-q tissue, luckily not a vein cuz that would hurt more since the needle and meds are replaced weekly. The initial dosing did nada but SHABAMMM! the second dose helped a lot!

I'm not nearly pain free, but I can handle it better and I'm grateful for the amount of "life" I've been given back. It's hard to explain, but for 2 months, every day I wondered how many more days I could take. So, the day-by-day mentality is what got me by as well as trying to focus on what I did have and could do rather than what I didn't or couldn't. Must admit that it crossed my mind a few times how many bottles of different narcotics were sitting at my bedside. Had it been another person, a person without so much support, a person who knows not how and when to seek professional help, a person in a deep depression, those pills could easily have done a person in, not the cancer. I guess no one tracks this stuff?

What the hell, I typed left hand only for 3 hours about this that and the other thing. I erased it!!!!! I can't repeat it, I don't want to. Well, now you know I can't use my right hand at all anymore, not even with the bionic arm! That's frustrating for sooooo many reasons, one being that blogging is a bitch now. But, much better than handwriting so I won't wallow in that for long.

The only thing I have to say is that where my entry left off, it seemed like I was pain free. Nope, not at all. The way I went on to describe it was like this: Instead of having 1 position be comfy on the couch, there are now several. I can do a few errands in a row if someone drives and holds doors and bags, but that gets me into a high level of pain which subsides after a while when I rest. So it's all about balancing need or desire with how much pain I'm willing to take. But if I pushed it past a few errands I'd likely end up in emerg again. So, my enthusiasm is all relative, but to me, right now, it makes a huuuuge difference in my quality of life.

Too bad so much got erased because I can only squeeze in one more entry before I start IL-2 in Buffalo on Monday. But we're leaving Sunday since I have to be at the hospital at the crack of dawn. I want to write about my feelings going into this treatment, many of which I've switched off for a while just so I can keep it together and get the most out of my days in waiting.

Blogging one handed is going to be a challenge going forward. Everything's a challenge these days. But I can handle 'em. One after the other, they keep rollin' in and the person I see in the mirror is not the one I knew 2.5 years ago, except for on the surface, and I'm certainly not talking physical surface. I'm different now. I just am.

posted by Sarah @ 11:57 PM   27 comments

BACK FROM ROUND 1

Jesus, what can I say? I feel like utter shit, I'm not gonna lie, but coming back to my blog and reading all your messages of encouragement bring tears to my eyes (my mom's helping out at home right now so I'm trying to hide the sobs – not time for the folks to know about this place yet) as I am reminded that soooo many angels are out there pulling and praying for me.

It's been so hard. IL-2 was better than expected the first week as some had told me it would be. My only symptoms were utter lethargy and drowsiness. None of the horrors I had read about. The torture was laying in that same bed, staring at that same wall, too mentally and physically tired to read magazines or play a game. I slept just to pass time. Sometimes I watched TV but most of the time the sound and action was too much for me to process so I kept it off. I feel shitty even complaining about that when people all over the world have hospital stays of months on end. But, it's how I felt, and I thought all the time of others who suffer the gambit of symptoms and I think I would have thrown myself out the window. I'm not that strong.

I received 9 out of the maximum of 14 doses possible in the week. They monitor you constantly to decide how much IL-2 you can take. Apparently, I took more doses than anyone else that week… so yay for me. I hope that means it'll work better, but then I also hope it works for everyone.

The real shittiness started at home. We left Buffalo Saturday morning and I have like 3 memories between then and Monday. Apparently the same male homecare nurse came to change my dressings (2 tumours on my arm and shoulder have raised thru the skin and are "draining" – yes, the site is horror flick worthy and it makes me feel disgusting times ten) on Sat, Sun & Mon, but I had no recollection of the first two visits so it was like meeting a new person on Monday. Monday was a bad day cuz that's when I started to get more lucid and aware of things, yet I was hallucinating a bit, but aware at the same time so I thought I was going crazy. That has been the worst part. When you think you may be crazy for the rest of your life, there are no words to describe the terror. One of my thoughts was that myself, Derek, my mom, my doctors were all characters in a board game and the IL-2 was one of the punishments. I so desperately wanted the game to end but there was no end. Yet, I was aware this made no sense and I must be hallucinating. Stuff like that was happening, along with a remarkable loss of speech, left hand strength (frustrating not being able to hold a glass with right or left hand!). It's Thursday now and I'm mainly just tired all the time, nauseous or constipated, headachy or dizzy, can't get comfy in bed cuz of my fat ass lymphedema arm and hand that can't be controlled anymore because of tumours blocking passage.... whaaa, whaaa, whaaa. Just general malaise and the depression is slipping in more too. It helps so much to hear your cheers and experiences though.

Nope, not all brave and stoic at all. I'm scared shitless to go back for round 2 on Monday. I was hoping to have a reprieve at home, but instead the symptoms started after I left. How many times have I cried, "I can't go back!"? Too many to count. But I will. Because so many others have and if they can do it, I can. And I can't refuse my best shot of a cure or at least a remission. How could I walk away from that? But I so fucking want to. I am scared out of my wits. I need to get back into focusing on the good and on the present. But my books that help so much are hard to read when I'm so tired and spinny. Derek offered to read to me, but the poor kid's life revolves around taking care of me now. He does EVERYTHING around the house, helps bathe me, dress me, sometimes helps in the bathroom, feeds me, has become my secretary and makes sure I take my pills. If I don't sleep (like last night), then neither does he, 'cept he has to work the next day. I hate depending on him so much. He's only 32, life is not supposed to be this way. But, it just plain is.

On a superfantastical surreal note, unbeknownst to me, my coworkers held a fundraiser for us so we didn't have to worry about the unpaid time Derek would take off work to come to Buffalo. They raised something like $7000! Oh, my God did I cry. My friend who organized [it] told me stories like of this one little girl of a coworker who when told of our situation told her mom she wanted to give all the money in her savings account to "that guy who has to take his sick wife to Buffalo". Her mom pointed out that was all her savings from birthdays and for education so maybe checking out the piggy bank would be more appropriate. She poured all the change on the bed and when asked how much she wanted to give she said, "Well, I'm six so I think I wanna give six dollars!" All that for us!!!! It is so bizarre to be the reason for a fundraiser, but the stories like that just make me want to fight more! There are too may people who care and I soooooooooo don't want to be a tragic story. Please God, give me strength.

Love to everyone! I'll update again after next treatment when I feel up to it.

posted by Sarah @ 12:20 PM   19 comments

REST IN PEACE, MY STRENGTH, MY ANGEL

Heather died. She actually died. Heather was my strength, I felt like she took me under her wing and encouraged me along the path. I knew she was doing badly. She lived in Buffalo and I was going to call her on the day she died, to see if somehow I might visit with her, even though she was bed ridden. But, I chickened out. I was afraid she'd be too sick, that we wouldn't be able to coordinate it anyway with me being in hospital. So, I guess her funeral must have been while I was in Buffalo. If I had known, I would have gone in a heartbeat.

I loved Heather, her wit, her will, her determination, and her constant ability to put her own woes aside and offer advice and an ear. I spoke with her once, around U.S. Thanksgiving. She said we were kindred spirits and I believe it. But Heather was 1000 times stronger and braver than I. Only 39 with 4 kids and a hubby, struggling financially and then with the beast. She was diagnosed the same day she gave birth to her last child not even 2 years ago. They noticed a suspicious mole on her leg as she was birthing. Unbelievably unfair. But, now she is a soaring angel, and as she was a huge part of my strength in life, she will remain so in death. I know that if Heather could do this thing, so can I.

Pleeeeease take time to read Heather's blog[22] from start (July) to finish. I guarantee you will never be so uplifted and inspired.

RIP March 2, 2007

posted by Sarah @ 1:36 PM   5 comments

---

22 *www.livingwithmelanoma.blogspot.com*

UPDATE BY DEREK

As you will all probably notice this is not Sarah's writing. This is her husband's attempt at an update, sorry no descriptive flowing prose, but blunt mis-spelled statements.

Sarah's [second] week in Buffalo (Mar 18 – 24) had its ups and its downs. Starting with the positive, she received 13 of 14 IL-2 doses, she showed an unbelievable ability to cope with a treatment that most can't handle very well. This is the reason why we're there, so we'll take as much as we can get. So understandably those kind of numbers mean swallowing some harsher, more prolonged side effects. These side effects appeared and took their toll and some still continue to linger, but I'm happy to say since today (Mar 28th) Sarah is feeling kinda normal, this is after a 7 day period of no solid food, a week and a half in bed with scary thoughts, hallucinations and confused states/dreams that melded with reality. It was really tough on her, questioning her own thoughts and working through them, separating real and the imagined. She did it, again just like last recovery, fought her drugged mind and won again.

She still cannot keep her food down and suffers from out of the blue massive headaches, but she speaks like her lovely self again, laughs, cries and lives like her self again. Her independence is on the horizon, her walking has improved and energy level is way better, still low but on the mend. I know she's had enough of my version of mothering and needs a break.

Sarah's one in a million, so strong and special it's beyond words. I realize a lot of you only know her through her blog, and this represents her well, but let me tell ya, the world has far too few people with Sarah's love, thoughtfulness and strength. Keep thinking of Sarah, she's a fighter and in the midst of a battle.

Derek

posted by Sarah @ 5:28 PM   61 comments

ANOTHER UPDATE BY DEREK

I'll just write a quick update now and I'll write more soon.

Sarah says hello to all and really wishes she could be the one giving the update.

Sarah's been in hospital for almost 4 weeks and during that time she's had surgery to remove the very large tumours that had broken through the skin on her arm and shoulder, they had become very infected. She has battled through some kidney problems and was almost put on dialysis (kidneys working perfectly again). She's finally started to feel better the last 3 or 4 days and there's also been an increase in her caloric intake and a slight movement towards solid food. All that said, she received some devastating news 2 days ago. The cancer has moved into her brain, 2 small metastasises were found on a CT scan. Radiation is still a good possibility, still waiting to talk to the radiologist. We're still fighting, yet understand what this means. It's a very sad time, but we live each moment, laughing and crying, and kissing and snuggling. Sarah's holding on tight and we'll make this road last and last, life is so sad but it's so good, everyday with my hero is a splendid one. Thanks for everybody's praying, and well wishes.

Right now we're focused on coming home. I'll update soon.

Derek

posted by Sarah @ 5:14 PM   63 comments

UNTITLED

Sarah's in rough shape. She received a week's worth of radiation to the head and a single dose to the right breast. No response. The last 2 days she's been in a drug induced sleep, the days previous to this involved periods of intense anxiety and pain, with few words to express herself.

It's so hard to write this next line. After fighting like no other, Sarah's going to die. Her [palliative care] Dr. thinks a few short days to a few short weeks. She's resting peacefully, but she must be in agony. I just hope she's OK and finds some long awaited peace and doesn't have to hear the C-word anymore. Wherever this place is, it will be much better off with Sarah in it. She's got lots more love to spread.

Safe travels my love.

DK

posted by Sarah @ 8:45 AM   207 comments

UNTITLED

Thanks for all the comments, I have read them and they are very touching.

Sarah's still fighting hard and has had miraculous periods of clarity, we've both said a lot of meaningful things to one another and for this I'm very grateful. Along with these moments of clarity are increasing episodes of delusion, confusion and hallucinations. These have become more prevalent over the last week. It's hard to see, handle and defuse. The disease in the brain is progressing but hopefully these symptoms will slow down since the latest flurry. She still assures me she's content and, when resting, is peaceful. The moments of clarity since the whole brain radiation will always be special, her (our) social worker says she's one of the special very few who are so strong and can regain so much function. To all her good friends, I've told her about all of your messages and e-mails. She knows she's loved and misses all. Most of the blog comments have also been read by Sarah. Thanks for all the support.

I'm really glad everyone understands how special Sarah is, I've truly never experienced such love, power and determination and her beauty remains, what a sight she is.

posted by Sarah @ 4:31 PM   90 comments

HOME VISIT...YEAH!

This entry was not posted on Sarah's blog, but it's an important part of her story, and demonstrates once again how strong and determined she was.

Sarah made it clear that she wanted to die at home, with the people, pets and things that she loved most. This was not to be.

When she was admitted to hospital April 21 for a "tune-up" to adjust her wonky blood levels, Sarah agreed with the understanding that she could have day passes to go home for a few hours anytime she wanted. However, she soon developed kidney disease, a side-effect from her IL-2 treatments, and she became gravely ill.

Sarah's team (oncologist, social worker, physical and occupational therapists) attempted to develop a plan so that Sarah could return home. But it quickly became apparent that the level of nursing care and equipment required was prohibitive.

However, in the last of several amazing turnarounds, on May 29 Sarah suddenly asked for lemonade. Subsequently, the periods of coherent conversations with Derek increased, and Sarah started eating a bit and exercising. She had a goal...to build enough strength for a visit home. What determination!

After several days of wheelchair tours around the hospital and surrounding grounds, the plan was set. The bus picked up Derek and Sarah in her special wheelchair at 11 am. Sarah's dad built a ramp so that she could get into the house. She toured her house, cuddled her beloved cats, and had a nap on her new comfy sofa (delivered only two days before admission to hospital). Sarah was so happy. I returned with her on the bus at 3 pm. Despite a wonderful driver, who drove very slowly, and took a longer but less bumpy route, the ride was excruciating. I honestly have no idea how Sarah remained conscious.

Upon return to the hospital, Sarah responded to all who asked, "It was awesome!"

inserted by Sarah's Mom

GOOD-BYE MY LOVE

Sarah Toller
February 7, 1977 – June 12, 2007

Sarah passed peacefully this morning with her mom and me by her side.

Now she rests, her love still radiating everywhere.

posted by Sarah @ 12:08 PM   292 comments

SARAH'S EULOGY

Good afternoon. I'm Mina and this is Liz and we've been best friends with Sarah since high school. We are deeply honoured that Sarah has asked us to help celebrate her life with all of you. We would like to share some of our favourite memories of our dear friend.

Anyone who knew Sarah, knew she was determined and was never afraid to go after what she wanted. One of our favourite stories is how she got Derek's attention which would later be referred to as the "Infamous Sweater Incident". After high school, Derek and Sarah both worked at Wal-Mart. She had been sweet on Derek for a few weeks, but wasn't having much luck. One night she deliberately left her sweater at Wal-Mart knowing Derek's shift ended later. Because Derek lived close to Sarah's mom's house she called him at work when she got home and asked if he could take her sweater home with him and she would come by his house to pick it up. Later that night she walked to his house to get her sweater and Derek invited her in for a drink. Her crafty plan had worked and the rest is history.

Another example of Sarah's determination was shared with us by her soccer team-mate and friend Abby. Abby and Sarah met when they both signed up to play for "Sisters in Soccer" in the summer of 2003. At the time, Abby had recently moved from New Zealand to London and didn't know very many people. Abby was really nervous to sign up as she hadn't played soccer before and didn't know anyone at registration. Coincidently, Sarah didn't know anyone either and they decided to put each others name down as the person they wanted to be on the same team with. This meant a lot to Abby because she was a friend before she was a friend and a friend when she didn't need to be. That is the person that Sarah was. The league was really social and they never took themselves too seriously. Abby played back in defence that year with Sarah, whom Abby described as a seasoned veteran, who played since age 3. Sarah had a powerful kick, and Abby always felt part of a force to be reckoned with when lining up beside Sarah to face the other team. Sarah definitely had skill and poise on the soccer field and looked good playing.

During one of the last games Sarah played in the second season, Abby and Sarah's team was losing pretty badly and for fun they decided to change it up a bit. So for the second half the forward positions played back and the back positions played forward, they had nothing to lose! Well, didn't Sarah go and score their team's only goal, to the dismay of the other team who thought they were so much better. Sarah and Abby's team still lost, but it was a sweet victory to get that one goal that denied the other team a shut out.

Sarah has also always had a sense of adventure! From junior kindergarten she was part of the French immersion program and in high school she had the opportunity to take some credits in France over the summer. Sarah and Derek both fell in love with Central America. They backpacked around Mexico for a few months together and later returned for another trip to Guatemala. Sarah brought us back Guatemalan worry dolls, which are supposed to take your worries away. Those dolls lived in Ecuador with Liz for a year and accompanied Mina to New Zealand, Australia and Thailand. Sarah also spent time in the rainforests of Costa Rica with her mom, drove the Cabot Trail with Liz in Cape Breton, travelled out West with Derek to visit their close friends in B.C., honeymooned in Bermuda as a wedding gift from Sarah's dad and walked the streets of Greenwich Village in New York City. Sarah's last travel adventure took her to England to visit an old university roommate, Lamia. Sarah explored the sites of London and took fabulous pictures of herself with the likes of Nelson Mandela, Brad Pitt and George Clooney at Madam Tussaud's Wax museum.

Sarah also lived her life with conviction and was very socially conscious. She loved animals, especially her adopted cats Misty and Mojo. Sarah made an effort in her life to eat a vegan diet and not buy leather products. Sarah also had a deep affection for children. She adored her nieces and nephews and dreamed of one day becoming a mother herself. Even when she was too sick to work, Sarah volunteered her time at a hospice and with children's programs to enrich her life and the lives of others.

During her illness, Sarah also became very vocal about patients' rights. She encouraged other women battling cancer to advocate for themselves and live life to the fullest. There were two women that Sarah worked with who also had been diagnosed with cancer and they instantly connected. It was a connection that is very difficult to explain to others who have never been on this particular journey in life. There were three of them in the office who started a club which they appropriately named the "C" Club and they would laugh about it because they certainly did not have people asking to join. They would go out for dinner on occasion and it was an evening out that they each looked forward to. They found a lot of support, humour, comfort and friendship by being together.

Sarah was one of the most resourceful people we have ever met. She could write anyone a resumé, find them a job, get them an apartment, decorate it, and re-vamp their wardrobe within 2 weeks and for under $100. Sarah planned her entire wedding from scratch using the internet and telephone. She designed a gorgeous wedding on a dime from the food to the decorations. Her mom, Pat, was her right hand lady throughout the execution of the day ensuring Sarah's detailed plans were carried out as she envisioned them. It was a beautiful July day in Derek's parent's backyard. The Kaskiw's put in countless hours of hard work ensuring their home and backyard looked perfect for the wedding. Sarah made a breath-taking bride and everyone there was honoured to take part in the celebration of Derek and Sarah's commitment to each other.

Shortly after she married Derek, Sarah fulfilled another one of her dreams, owning her own home. They moved into a house on Empress Ave. Her eye for decor and sense of style combined with her dad's carpentry skills turned it into a home that Sarah and Derek were very proud of. Sarah hosted several creative get-togethers at their home including a vegan croquet party and last year held a Christmas exchange for 20 of her and Derek's closest friends.

Sarah was undeniably a wonderful friend. When a co-worker was going through a tough time, Sarah could tell something was wrong. One day she casually walked by her co-worker's desk and put a stick-it note on her computer, and continued on her way without saying a word. Her co-worker looked at the piece of paper to see a big happy face and note saying "I thought you might need a smile today". Well it worked. When she went to thank Sarah for cheering her up, Sarah told her to keep it with her as a sign that would always be there. From that day on, her co-worker knew that she could always count on Sarah to cheer her up ... simply with one of her big radiant smiles.

She talked us through lost jobs, break-ups, family drama and very bad haircuts. Sarah always took the time to make important occasions special. She was always the one who remembered our birthdays. Each year she would call us to remind us when the other one's was. Not a year went by that we didn't receive a card. Last year for my birthday Sarah arranged for the 3 of us to get glammed up with MAC Makeovers and go out for dinner. None of us wears too much make-up so we asked the MAC girls to take it easy on us. Our MAC Makeovers lasted a total of 5 minutes each. Sarah came out looking fantastic, but unfortunately Mina and I looked like someone had taken a marker and drawn on our faces. Sarah was so excited and she loved it so much that we didn't have the heart to tell her we didn't like it. On the way to the restaurant, Mina and I took turns secretly whipping the make-up off hoping she wouldn't notice. By the time we got to the restaurant we had wiped most of it off and Sarah was not too pleased. Regardless, it was a wonderful and memorable day. The three of us always had a great time together whether we were having a tea, a drink on her deck, or out on the town. She was a true friend.

If you could get Sarah out she was so much fun to be around. She always claimed to hate dancing, but after a few drinks she was the first person on the dance floor and the last to leave. We obtained a little more evidence of this from Sarah's long term friend Amy.

When Sarah was younger, it was a long time tradition that her mom would take her and Amy to the Western fair. When the year came that they were able to go alone, they also went to their first outdoor concert which was Tom Cochrane's "Life is a Highway" tour. They began watching the concert in the bleachers until Sarah decided she wanted to get closer, so they jumped the wall and went closer to the stage. Not long after that it began to pour rain. Sarah started to dance in the mud, then Amy joined in, and they danced like that for the rest of the concert. By the end of it they were soaked from the rain and covered in mud.

Another adventure that Sarah and Amy had was the year Sarah first got her license and some how convinced her mother to lend her new blue Mazda to go camping. The trip should have taken them an hour, but ended up taking 2½ hours. When they arrived, it was not what they were expecting. It was a campground that was literally in the middle of a corn field, run by bikers who had a carefree philosophy like hippies. But, they made the most of it by dancing to live bands playing in the campground until 5:00 in the morning.

It is not Liz's or my intention to focus on the cancer, but we think it is important to recognize what Sarah's journey has taught us over these last 3 years. From Sarah we learned a great deal about strength. People would always ask Sarah "How do you deal with it?" and her reply would always be the same: "You just do". Her ability to be strong for not only herself, but also for her family and friends was a true testament to her inner strength. She made it so easy for all of us. If anything, Sarah has taught us that everyone is strong and that you can face things you never thought possible. To doubt that you could face anything considering what she went through would be an injustice to her struggle against cancer. We owe it to ourselves to know that we can get through almost anything.

Courage, like strength, Sarah had an abundance of. The courage to be weak, to be sad, to be happy, to be at peace and to find humour in even the most devastating of situations. A true test of courage is fighting a battle you know you may lose, but Sarah never wavered from her goal to live.

We learned about what friendship really means, that it is the little things, the big things, it's about sticking with it even if you're scared and sticking it out with someone you love because there is more going on than yourself.

We learned the importance of letting people in, and letting people let you in, even if it is uncomfortable. It is so worth it.

Finally, we learned the true meaning of devotion and unconditional true love. If anyone in this room has ever doubted that true love exists… it does… in its purest form with Sarah and Derek.

We would like to thank Pat, John [Sarah's dad], and Bryan [Sarah's brother] for loving Sarah so much. Pat, we have cherished the time we've spent getting to know you over the past few months.

Derek, your love for Sarah is truly an amazing blessing. Sarah was able to draw from your strength and courage. You were her hero as much as she was yours.

Finally, we would like to thank Sarah for giving us the greatest gift of friendship. We simply love you and you will be greatly missed…

Thank you.

Love you Sarah xoxoxoxoxoxoxoxxo

> *posted by Sarah @ 4:20 PM   42 comments*

EPILOGUE

The following is excerpted from *http://doubleagentgirl.spaces. live.com/*.

JULY 05, 2007 –
CANCER – SARAH TOLLER AND DIVINE INTERVENTION

I have just understood the magnitude of something that has happened to me recently. I don't ever want to forget the crippling indebtedness that I have to a stranger I never met – Sarah Toller.

Back in April, I had a strange conversation with someone at my volunteer job. For all of you who don't know what I do, I volunteer in a child minding room at a local gym – where I had this offhand conversation with a child's parent and her friend. I honestly don't remember how it came up – especially since I'm not prone to discussing personal physical anomalies with virtual strangers – but this time I did.

Off hand, I mentioned to this woman (referred to as "S") that I had a strange mole inside my bellybutton. This mole had first been noticed by me five years ago while I was pregnant with Taylor. As all mothers know, your bellybutton has a tendency to turn itself out in the late stages. Mine only partially did, which is when I noticed a TINY little freckle – which I first thought was dirt. LOL. I noticed around three or four months before this conversation, in the shower, that this mole was now the size of a pencil eraser. I thought it odd, and then spoke to S about it.

Let me say, S is not a nurse, or a health care professional. Why I should choose her is irrational – but prophetic.

S mentioned that her sister-in-law was battling skin cancer (melanoma) that resulted from a mole. This is Sarah Toller. She was diagnosed with stage 3 melanoma from this mole at the age of 27. (oddly – my age presently). S and her friend K strongly recommended that I see a dermatologist about this mole as soon as I can. They certainly stressed the importance of SOON.

And so – I did. I made an appointment, and in May the dermatologist opted to remove the mole in its entirety right there in the office and send it away for biopsy. I was sent home with a few stitches and an appointment four weeks later for the results. Of course, I worried, I thought about what cancer would mean for me, my children, our lives...

On June 12, I returned to the dermatologist for the results. Turns out – it was cancer – HOWEVER – it had NOT spread outside the mole. So – since they had removed the mole and surrounding tissue – it's no longer a problem for me. I need to follow up every six months to have all other moles checked – but no further treatment is necessary. Of course – I am grateful to S for the recommendation.

Today is the first time that I have seen S since this whole thing started – school has kept me away from volunteering as much as I had, so I took this opportunity to express to S my gratitude.

S burst into tears. Her sister-in-law, Sarah Toller, had lost her battle with melanoma, and passed away almost a month ago. She hugged me, we chatted about my "luck" – I thanked her for her intervention. S mentioned that Sarah Toller had actually kept an online blog through her struggle with the disease. She thought I may like to read it – and passed the link on to me. So this afternoon when I got home, I opened the link and began to read the entries Sarah made over the course of one year – documenting her battle with cancer.

What a brave woman. She was so positive; she fought so hard, she BELIEVED she was going to beat it! I laughed, I cried, I struggled for breath between sobs in the final entries, made by her husband in the last weeks of Sarah Toller's struggle. Then I read her eulogy.

Now – I am grateful first to Sarah Toller. Without her push for awareness, and her battle for her life – S would never have been so adamant in her recommendations to me. I believe Sarah wanted people to know – early diagnosis cures 90% of melanomas. Sadly, she died the day I was saved – and I cannot help but think – some forces were at work to bring me to this stranger S, who passed on a tidbit of information that led me to this hero Sarah Toller – whose death – probably saved my life. Rest in Peace.

Amanda Karr is currently an English Major at the University of Western Ontario, single mother of two and part-time volunteer and peer tutor.

S, as referred to in Amanda's blog, is Sarah Cartwright, Sarah Toller's sister-in-law. She lives in London, Ontario, with her husband and three young boys. Without her astute insight and intervention, Amanda's story may have not turned out so happily.

A WORD OF CAUTION
FROM DR. W. GIFFORD-JONES

Each year in North America one person dies every hour due to a malignant melanoma. So what can you do to protect yourself? And how much should we shield ourselves from the sun?

It's prudent to do a mole check of your whole body at regular intervals. But it's not easy to examine your own back. So if you have a partner, check each other's back from time to time.

What do you look for when examining the skin? Melanomas come in a variety of colours. Some are coal black, some darker around the outside of the mole. Still others contain a mixture of white, purple, blue and red. And some are the shade of skin.

Nearly all dangerous moles have irregular or indefinite margins. A red inflamed area is often present around the periphery of the mole and in some cases there may be satellite moles in the immediate vicinity.

A red light should flash in your head if a mole develops a tingling sensation or becomes itchy, grows larger, tender, ulcerated and bleeds easily. See your doctor immediately if there's the slightest suspicion that an innocent mole is changing in any way.

There's an old surgical saying, "when in doubt, cut it out." No doctor, of course, wants to remove a normal appendix. But it does no harm if a suspicious mole is removed, then found later to be normal.

Protect yourself from the sun. As Rudyard Kipling wrote, "Only mad dogs and Englishmen go out in the noon day sun." Too much sun exposure is a major cause of many melanomas. However, don't go to the other extreme and become paranoid about the sun. Recent research indicates that some sunlight might even help to protect against melanomas.

We have also known for years that sunlight stimulates the production of vitamin D, a vitamin crucial to bone health and the prevention of osteoporosis. There's also evidence that vitamin D may play a role in preventing colon cancer.

The message of this research does not mean we can all go out and bake in the sun. Rather, as in most situations in life, moderation is the best choice.

So how much sun exposure is needed? Experts suggest about 30 minutes a day. But in Canada and the northern U.S. we receive no benefit from the sun from October to February. It's therefore prudent to take 800 units of vitamin D daily during these months.

Dr. W. Gifford-Jones was educated at the University of Toronto and Harvard Medical School. He is the author of seven books and his syndicated medical column, *The Doctor Game,* appears in over 100 newspapers across Canada and the United States. He has a medical practice in Toronto. For more information and for weekly medical tips, visit his website *www.mydoctor.ca/gifford-jones.*

FURTHER INFORMATION AND SUPPORT

BOOKS

Kaufmann, Howard L. *The Melanoma Book: A Complete Guide to Prevention and Treatment, Including the Early Detection Self-Exam Body Map.* Gotham Books, a division of Penguin Group (USA), Inc., New York, New York.

Tolle, Eckhart. *The Power of Now. A Guide to Spiritual Enlightenment.* Namaste Publishing Inc., Vancouver, British Columbia.

Wilber, Ken. *Grace and Grit, Spirituality and Healing in the Life and Death of Treya Killam Wilber.* Shambhala Publications, Inc., Boston, Massachusetts.

AVAILABLE ON THE INTERNET

The *Canadian Cancer Society* is a "national, community-based organization of volunteers, whose mission is the eradication of cancer and the enhancement of the quality of life of people living with cancer." See their website for locations and further information. *www.cancer.ca*

Canadian Melanoma Foundation – *www.derm.ubc.ca/division/cmf/cmf1.htm*

Canadian Skin Cancer Foundation – *www.canadianskincancer.com/melanoma.html*

Cancer Care Ontario – *www.cancercare.on.ca/english/home/*

Melanoma Patient's Information Page at *www.mpip.org*, provides support and information on-line for those who want to be a proactive participant in their treatment decisions.

Melanoma Center at *www.melanomacenter.org* provides an excellent introduction to the risks, prevention, detection, diagnosis, staging, treatment and living with melanoma. It also has an extensive "related links" page for those who want to be a proactive participant in their treatment decisions.

Melanoma Research Foundation, *www.melanoma.org/*, is another excellent U.S. website.

National Cancer Institute at *www.cancer.gov/* is loaded with information about all cancers, including treatment, prevention, screening, genetics, causes, clinical trials and how to cope with cancer. Note this is a U.S. organization, and therefore all treatments described may not be available in Canada.

National Cancer Institute of Canada, *www.ncic.cancer.ca*, is Canada's premier research organization. This website contains Canadian cancer statistics and information on various current research projects.

Radiation Therapy and You is an e-book of interest to those about to get, or are getting radiation therapy, and their caregivers. It is available free on-line at *www.cancer.gov/cancertopics/radiation-therapy-and-you/*

Real Time Cancer, *www.realtimecancer.org/default.asp,* is a Canadian website focused on educating and supporting young adults. Includes articles, online discussions and much more.

Wellspring, a Canadian network of cancer support centres. See their website for locations and specific services:
www.wellspring.ca

ABBREVIATIONS AND DEFINITIONS

adjuvant	treatment following surgery
axilla	armpit; more particularly the cavity beneath the junction of the arm or anterior appendage and shoulder or pectoral girdle containing the axillary artery and vein, a part of the brachial plexus of nerves, many lymph nodes, and fat and areolar tissue
cm	centimetre
CT	Computerized Tomography (as in CT scan)
INF	interferon
IL-2	a specific Interleukin treatment
mel	melanoma
mets	metastases
mm	millimetre or malignant melanoma
MPIP	Melanoma Patients Information Page (*www.mpip.org*)
NCI	National Cancer Institute
NIH	National Institutes of Health
NED	No Evidence of Disease
MRI	Magnetic Resonance Imaging
onc	oncologist

OR operating room
(also used to refer to an operation itself)

path pathology, as in "path report" and "path results". Refers to "*the anatomic and physiological deviations from the normal that constitute
disease or characterize a particular disease*", as
defined by Merriam-Webster

PET Positron Emission Tomography

Perioperative relating to, occurring in, or being the period
around the time of a surgical operation

PMH Princess Margaret Hospital (Toronto)

Sub-q Subcutaneous (refers to tumours, injection
sites, or other, depending on context)

WLE Wide Local Excision

ABOUT THE AUTHOR

Sarah Lynne Toller was born February 7, 1977 in Ottawa, Ontario. When she was 2 years old, she moved with her family to London, Ontario, where she grew up.

Sarah had no time for her younger brother, Bryan, and would regularly chase him around the house, and beat him up when she had the opportunity. Her mom often reminded her that one day he would grow to be bigger than her and would get his revenge. By adolescence, Sarah came to see her brother as less of a threat and more as a younger brother to look after. In fact, Sarah grew to be 5' 6", and Bryan reached 6' 4".

Sarah's early school years were fun-filled and happy. She attended French Immersion, enjoyed soccer, swimming, riding her bicycle, and had many close friends and playmates. Her backyard was the neighbourhood playground.

Sarah was 12 years old when her parents separated, and her world fell apart. While she managed to maintain reasonable grades in school (with the help of summer school), she expanded her circle of friends and activities to include some not approved by her parents. She had several difficult and painful experiences during her teen years, which she ultimately handled with an amazing maturity. Despite some emotional scars, Sarah turned herself around to become an advocate for those in need.

Sarah became an adult the day she left home and moved to Toronto to attend university. At her parents' insistence, she endured residence her first year, but then happily enjoyed sharing various accommodations with different housemates for her remaining years in Toronto. Sarah worked hard at numerous part-time jobs to maintain her stylish wardrobe.

By the time she graduated, she was ready to return to London, with her love Derek. They were truly living the "happily-ever-after" story when she was diagnosed with malignant melanoma in 2004.

In this book, a transcription of her blog, she tells the rest of her story.